MW00960186

ASIAN HERBS
and their wondrous health-giving properties

SUDHIR AHLUWALIA

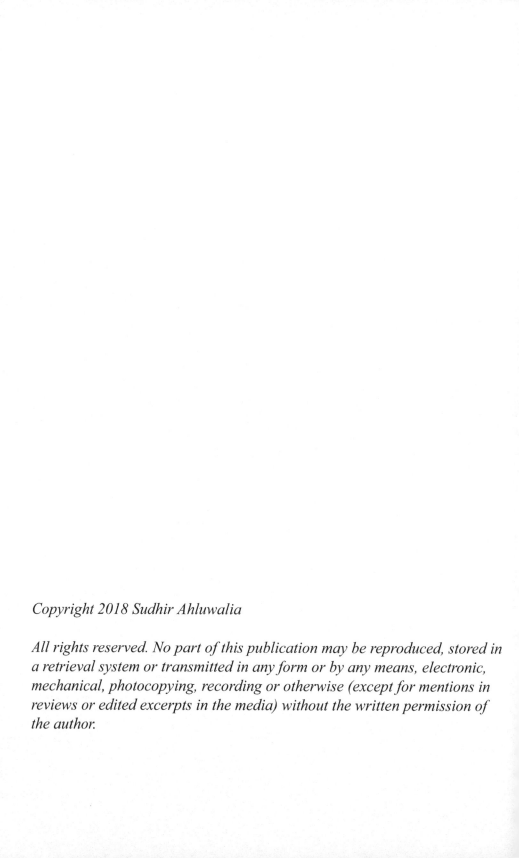

Copyright 2018 Sudhir Ahluwalia

All rights reserved. No part of this publication may be reproduced, stored in a retrieval system or transmitted in any form or by any means, electronic, mechanical, photocopying, recording or otherwise (except for mentions in reviews or edited excerpts in the media) without the written permission of the author.

About the Author

Sudhir Ahluwalia has been a member of the Indian Forest Service, global head of business consulting group in Tata Consultancy Services, business advisor to multiple companies and now an author and columnist. His writing is largely focused on herbs and natural products.

His other book titles include- *Holy Herbs: Modern Connections to Ancient Plants, Natural Solutions for Cancer - Amazing cancer healing properties from nature.*

All his titles are available on Amazon.

His webpage is www. sudhirahluwalia.com.,

DISCLAIMER

The purpose of this book is to provide information. None of the information provided in this book is intended as medical advice. Always seek advice from medical professionals before starting any treatments.

DEDICATION

This book is dedicated to
Vibha, my wife, partner
and friend for close to forty years.

ACKNOWLEDGEMENTS

A special thanks to Dr. Ravikumar Senior Botanist, Foundations of Revitalization of Local Health Traditions, India who was kind enough to share pictures of various plants and trees mentioned in the book. A special thanks to D.K,Ved, School Advisor, School of Conservation and Natural Resources, TransDisciplinary University, India who is also my friend, colleague and probably the best known medicinal plant expert in India.

PRE – RELEASE REVIEWS

As a botanist, I found the discussion on the botanical aspects of various Asian plants is interesting and meticulously described. The author has also comprehensively addressed the historical, medicinal and industrial uses of herbs, shrubs and trees.

Dr Ravikumar, Senior Botanist, FRLHT, Bengaluru, India

The author did a great job outlining the major parts of Ayurveda medicine and plants. His methods of delivery are very clear and very useful.

Aditya Kumar, Founder Smart Cube

Sudhir Ahluwalia represents a very interesting blend of history of Asian herbs, modern applications, such as current uses as a food and medicine, as well as outlook presenting likely future developments. While Asian herbs are the major focus of the book, surprisingly many additional relevant and exciting aspects are also discussed, ranging from the increasingly recognized regulatory role of microbiota for the human health, to emerging applications of 3D bioprinting.

Atanas Atanasov, Professor and Head of Microbiology, Institute of Genetics and Animal Breeding, IGHZ, Poland

The book 'Asian Herbs' written by Dr Sudhir Ahluwalia, ex senior IFS officer & business consulting head of Tata Consultancy Services gives a very nice information along with colored photographs and a very vivid description about the common herbs used in India & China for pharmacological and culinary uses.

The book not only dwells on the historical & mythological importance of the herbs but also their geographic distribution, morphology, alkaloids found in them, their pharmacological & culinary uses, results of different authentic research done on them in the important research institutions of the world with their references. This kind of perfection is very rarely found in the related literature found scattered here & there. I hope this book will be a great asset for the students, research scholars and the people engaged in the pharmacological & culinary fields.

I heartily congratulate Dr Sudhir Ahluwalia for all the painstaking efforts which he has put into bringing out this masterpiece treatise on the chosen subject.

Jyoti Swaroop Asthana, IFS (Retd)
Ex Principal Chief Conservator of Forests
& Head of Forest Force, UP, Lucknow, India

TABLE OF CONTENTS

Sudhir Ahluwalia

INTRODUCTION

This is a book that seeks to provide a holistic view of the world of Asian herbs. Select herbs and trees from India and China are subjected to critical analysis through a review of the history, botany, ecology, trade, medicinal, and other uses of each of them. Herbs, trees, and shrubs are sources of human food, shelter, medicine, and security. The trend to use plants as food, for taste, as preservatives, in medicine, and in manufacturing of industrial and other products continues from ancient times.

Herbs have been a source of perfumes, incense, and cosmetics too. Perfume makers are said to have operated in the Palace of Mari, in what is today Tel Hariri, in Syria and in Mesopotamia as early as 1800 BC. Archeological evidence in support of this use has also been uncovered in other parts of the world.

There are references to herbs in nearly every ancient religious and secular literature in the world. Nature was an integral part of ancient society. This book draws upon references on herbs from the Bible, Koran, Greek, Egyptian, Mesopotamian, Hindu, and Zorastrian literature.

The use of herbs, plants, and spices in Ayurveda has been extensively documented. Sushruta samhita and Charakasamhita are two major medicinal ancient compilations of India. These were written by Sushruta and Charaka, two of ancient India's most renowned surgeons. These contain a compilation of medicinal practices that were in use from the period between 6th century BC and 5th century AD.

The earliest references to herbs used in China go back to the time of Sheng Nung around 28th century BC (Encyclopedia Britannica). The Chinese have been using cinnamon, aloe vera, cloves, tea, alfafa, and ginger in the treatment for many ailments.

1

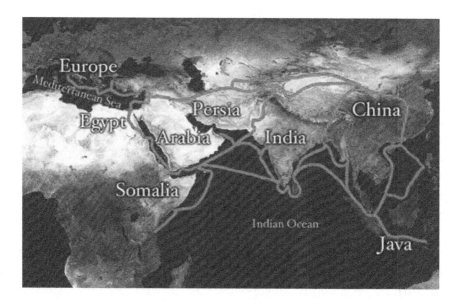

Picture 1: Ancient Spice Routes
The Silk Road route is shown in red Trade

Herbs and spices were highly valued commodities in ancient times. Ancient trans-civilization trade in these products used three transcontinental trade routes—the Incense Route, the Spice Route, and the Silk Road.
The Incense Route connected the Mediterranean region to the Land of Punt in Africa and Arabia. This trade route is said to have been used extensively to bring goods from Africa to Ancient Egypt, Greece, and later into Rome from around 700 BC to 200 AD.

The Spice Route connected India and Southeast Asia in the East to the Mediterranean centers of Rome, Greece, and Egypt in the West. The route was used to transport pepper, cardamom, cinnamon, nutmeg, cloves, wood, ghee (clarified butter), cloth, and metal tools from India, Sri Lanka, and the region around modern-day Indonesia.

The third major ancient transport route was the Silk Road that connected Europe and China through Persia, Central Asia, and via Tibet to India.

Herbal Industry Overview

Herbs are an invaluable gene pool resource. This resource has played an important role in the development of agriculture, natural sciences, drug discovery, and plant disease management. Modern drugs, though, are in most cases chemical-based.

According to Global Industry Analysts, a market research firm, the global herbal supplements and remedies market was estimated to reach $107 billion by the year 2017.
Herbal products often face a supply shortage with demand outstripping supply. Often, the supply shortage is due to ecological deterioration of the ecosystems caused by overexploitation and biotic pressures from cattle grazing.

Cultivation is the most common mode adopted to meet demand. This option is not available for species that can only be collected from the wild (examples Terminalia bellerica, Tinospora cordifolia etc.). Cultivation practices for these have not been developed yet. However, the herbs and plants selected for detailed study and analysis in this book are all cultivatable.

Herbal supplements are quite popular in Europe and the US. There is a vibrant market for these products in these regions. But it is India and China that are showing the fastest year-on-year growth of herbal products. In countries such as France, Germany, UK, and India, herbal supplements are retailed along with pharmaceuticals in drugstores. In the US, the sale of herbal medicine is not permitted.

The natural products industry, though, is not restricted to herbs, shrubs, and trees. Microbiota (microorganisms found in the gut) form another increasingly important component of this industry. Programs like the Human Microbiome Project[1] are leading to better understanding of the microorganisms living in the gut. Some of the breakthrough innovation in this space has led to a spurt in demand for microflora-based natural food products.

As the connection between gut microbiota and the human diet has become better understood, scientists and physicians have started recommending diets that support growth of gut microbiota. Justin and Erica Sonnenburg, in their 2015 book, The Good Gut, have prescribed a seven-day "Microbiota Friendly" diet for North Americans, a diet rich in fiber.

The importance of probiotic bacteria in human digestion is now universally accepted. Physicians commonly recommend probiotic foods to assist in the treatment of a variety of ailments. Probiotic yoghurts and other fermented foods that help build gut microbiota are becoming increasingly popular. Today, these are getting fully integrated into the healthy food consumption basket.

Debate on Efficacy of Herbal Products

The world in general is not yet convinced of the claimed efficacy of herbal products as medication.
Herbal medical science is still regarded with a lot of suspicion, although there are dedicated followers of Ayurveda, traditional Chinese and Tibetan medicine, Unani, and other niche plant-based medicine systems.

The regulators across the world too—and this includes USFDA—are unconvinced about the claimed medicinal value of herbs to the extent that there is hardly one that has agreed to certify herbal medicine. Herbal products, in most parts of the world, are approved for sale as nutraceuticals only.

---

1   The Human Microbiome Project (HMP) was launched in 2008. It is an extension of another ambitious global project—the Human Genome Project. HMP seeks to understand the metagenome (the combined genomes of all the microbes) of 300 healthy people. Five body areas are being sampled: skin, mouth, nose, colon, and vagina.

Some herbal product companies are particularly keen to obtain scientific support for claims of efficacy of their products to expand their customer base beyond traditional herbal enthusiasts.

In this quest, companies have entered into alliances with reputed research institutions. This has led to a lot of experimentation and publishing on company-specific products. This literature forms part of the business development collateral for these companies.

Overall, the herbal industry is largely dominated by small- and medium-sized companies. The market share of the herbal product industry in the healthcare industry continues to be small.

Trials and Testing

The biggest impediment to development of science–backed, natural-product medicine is the difficulty faced in conducting animal and human trials. Unlike doctors of modern medicine, practitioners of herbal medicine recommend products that contain a combination of herbs. Many of the popular herbal products could contain a dozen or more herbs and minerals. These products are often based on ancient herbal medicine formulations.

The molecule concentration in plants is rarely uniform. These are known to vary with strain, species, geographic distribution, type of soil, and cultivation practices. These variations add to the complication in creating a replicable identical that can undergo a modern clinical testing acceptable to a regulator.

The availability of suitable subjects to conduct a double placebo human trial is another impediment. All these barriers make natural products manufacturers wary of launching human trials. Further, conducting a human trial is a complicated, time consuming, and expensive affair.

These days, testing gets disrupted because of scientific success in developing live human tissue through bioprinting using 3D bioprinters. This makes it possible for scientists to conduct trials on human tissue safely with no ethical or cultural implications.

The use of 3D bioprinters and live tissue modeling has led to a rise in demand for 3D cell tissue. According to BCC Research, a market research agency, the demand for this tissue is estimated to reach $2.2 billion by 2019. It is a three-dimensional tissue model that lies at the heart of bioprinting.

Tissue modeling work is largely being done by research institutions. For instance, Johns Hopkins Bloomberg School of Public Health has created a mini brain organoid all with neurons and other critical cellular compositions of the human brain.

3D printing of living tissue could begin on an industrial scale as early as the next decade. This will give a huge boost to pre-clinical drug and other material testing on live human tissue. Other applications will emerge in time.

Some of the bigger pharmaceutical, biotech, and cosmetic manufacturers have begun leveraging this technology to test[2] their products. BASF, the German company, has also entered into an agreement with a French biotech company that is into bioprinting tissue.

BASF will use this technology to improve their skin model, "Mimeskin." This is claimed to be the closest equivalent to the original physiological tissue of the human skin.

---

2   On April 1, 2015, Organovo Holding, a US-based 3D bioprinter and tissue modeling company, entered into an agreement with L'Oréal USA Products, Inc. They agreed to collaborate on developing skin tissue models using a bioprinting platform. L'Oréal was to use this in the development, manufacturing, testing, evaluation, and sale of non-prescription cosmetics, beauty, dermatology, and skin-care products and nutraceutical supplements.

It is important to note that the agreement between L'Oréal and Organovo includes testing of nutraceutical formulations. The deal between Nestlé and L'Oréal and other similar deals indicate that going forward, 3D bioprinted human tissue will be used to test nutraceutical formulations. This should open the way for the use of this technology by manufacturers of natural products too. Disruptive technology may finally be breaking into this industry.

While the debate on advancements in technology and the subsequent scientific support available to herbal products continues, there does exist in the minds of many people the desire to better understand the properties of major herbs and plants in everyday use by humans. We will now turn our attention towards some of the major Asian herbs in depth.

Herbs are increasingly being looked at as a source of new drugs. Drug discovery from chemical sources is becoming more and more difficult. The cost of discovery is also rising, leading to this shift back to natural products.

The popularity of organic and herbal food, herbal beauty care, and medicinal products is rising. This is spurred on the back of a general belief that herbal solutions have little to no side effects. This is despite the questions on quality control and good manufacturing practices in the natural products industry that continue to be raised by both consumers and regulators.

This book includes a review of the current state of scientific research on

The chapters of the book are summarized below:

Chapter 1: The history of herbs and herbal trade

India and China are home to many of most popular herbs and spices in use in food and medicine across the world. These commodities were actively traded in ancient times, and cultural interaction based on them goes back to 3rdmillennium BC. This continues today too.

Chapter 2: Globally used Aromatic Plants from India

India is home to many aromatic trees, shrubs, and herbs. Aromatic plants have been in use since the earliest of times in places of worship, in medicine, and to make beauty and industrial products.

Three very important aromatic plants are detailed in this chapter. These are sandalwood (Santalum album), camphor (Cinnamomum camphora), and holy basil (Ocimum basilicum). Sandalwood and camphor were actively traded commodities in history. Sandalwood continues to be traded even today.

Chapter 3: Indian sacred trees with amazing health-giving properties

Sacred trees were integral to Shamanic, Hindu, Egyptian, Sumerian, Toltec, Mayan, Norse, Celtic, and Christian traditions. Parallels between Eastern and Western traditions on sacredness of trees are drawn in this chapter. We will also peek at the folkloric references to each of the trees mentioned in the ancient Hindu texts.

Papal (Ficus religiosa), Banyan (Ficus benghalensis), Wood Apple (Aegle marmelos), Kadamba (Anthocephalus cadamba),Ashoka (Saraca indica), Rudraraksha (Elaeocarpus ganitrus), Mango (Mangifera indica), and Neem (Azadirachta indica) are the tree species reviewed in this chapter.

Chapter 4: Spices of India

Indian cuisine is known for its prolific use of spices. Sweet, sour, salty, spicy, bitter, and astringent are the six tastes listed in literature on Indian cuisine. A well-balanced Indian meal takes care to contain all six tastes.

Some of the common traditional local spices described in the chapter are turmeric, cloves, Indian bay leaf, and cardamom.

Chapter 5: Herbs and Spices of China

Herbs and spices are integral to Chinese food and medicine. Eating the right food helps in maintaining nutritional well-being and helps heal a sick body. This chapter examines select herbs in popular use in Chinese cuisine. These are garlic (Allium sativum), onion (Allium cepa), ginger (Zingiber officinale), Star anise (Illicium verum), Sichuan pepper (Zanthoxylum sps), Fennel (Foeniculum vulgare), and clove (Syzygium aromaticum)

Chapter 6: Marijuana, fiber, intoxicant and medicine

Hemp is one of the earliest agricultural crops known to man (Sagan, 1977). The plant was valued for its fiber and in medicine. There are references to marijuana in the Chinese pharmacopeia, going back to 1500 BC (National Institute of Drug Abuse - Marijuana Research Findings - 1976, 1977). The use of cannabis in India can be traced back to Vedic times. Marijuana is regarded as a recognized medicine in the 3rd edition of the US Pharmacopoeia under the name of Extractum Cannabis or Extract of Hemp and was listed until 1942.

This chapter looks at the scientific evidence in support and against the use of marijuana in medicine and as a recreational drug.

Chapter 7: Ginseng research supported medicinal properties

Ginseng has been in use in Chinese medicine for millennia. Ginseng comes from the fleshy roots of perennial slow-growing plants belonging to eleven species and two genera. Panax ginseng is the most common of the ginseng yielding plants. A detailed review of ginseng is conducted in this chapter.

CHAPTER 1

History of herbs and herbal trade

The Indus Valley Civilization is the earliest documented civilization of South Asia. The civilization settlements covered most parts of Northwestern India, modern day Pakistan, and extends west into the eastern parts of Afghanistan. This civilization is said to have flourished from 2600 BC to 1800 BC. Prior to this period, settlements were possibly in the form of small, widely-dispersed clusters.

Some of the cities of this civilization have been excavated by archaeologists, the most prominent being in Harappa and Mohenjo Daro located in Punjab and Sindh provinces of modern day Pakistan. Studies conducted by Arunima Kashyap and Steve Weber at Farmana, an Indus Valley Civilization burial site close to Delhi, found traces of turmeric, ginger, and garlic in pots recovered from the site (Weber et al., 2011).

Jane McIntosh's studies reveal that the Harappans consumed mustard, coriander, mango, caper, garlic, turmeric, ginger, cumin, and cinnamon. Sesame and probably linseed oil were used in cooking. Grinding stones used to pound grain and spices have been excavated from these settlements (McIntosh, 2008).

Mesopotamia was a major civilization neighboring the Indus Valley. Mesopotamia had a thriving agriculture, but little wood and virtually no maritime tradition. The Indus Valley people, on the other hand, were mariners. They traded extensively in wood, gemstones, spices, and exotic animals. (Ratnagar, 2001).

The Mesopotamians called the Indus Valley people "Meluha" or the Dark People (Ratnagar, 2001). Mesopotamian tablets mention boats from Meluha docking in their ports. Archaelogical evidence that prove the existence of this ancient trade has been uncovered from sites in modern day Oman, Bahrain, and Iran.

Ancient Egypt and Greece

Hieroglyphs from the time of Queen Hatshepsut of Egypt circa 1508 BC show prevalent use of cassia, cinnamon, myrrh, and frankincense. Cassia was imported from China via the Silk Road, and cinnamon came from India. Myrrh and frankincense were brought into Ancient Egypt from neighboring North and Northeast Africa.

Trade was and still is influenced by geopolitical conditions prevailing during a period. Greece, Egypt, Persia, Assyria, Rome, India, and China traded sporadically over the millennia. Wars, strife, and political uncertainty affected trade and availability of goods.

Egypt was conquered by the Assyrians in the 7th century BC. This opened the land route to Egypt from Asia via Mesopotamia. Maritime routes were more popular. Trade in the Mediterranean region was conducted mainly by the Phoenicians in ships made of cedar wood.

China

In China, the earliest records on herbs can be traced back to Shen Nung (circa 2695 BC) who is regarded as the Father of Chinese medicine. It is said that Nung identified characteristics of herbs by tasting them. He is said to have tasted 365 herbs before dying from a toxic overdose of one (On Herbal Medical Experiment Poisons - Shen Nung c. 27th cent. BC). Shen Nung's work forms the basis of traditional Chinese medicine.

Chinese tradition has it that individual organs and body functions, indeed, all things in the universe, are interconnected. The body is influenced by the ecosystem surrounding it. This is based on principles enunciated in Taoism— the ancient Chinese way of life. Disharmony leads to disbalance and disease. Herbs are used to correct disharmony.

Asian Herbs

The Maluku Islands were major producer of cloves, nutmeg, and mace. There existed an active ancient maritime trade between the Chinese Han Empires and the people of Malacca (Maluku). Cloves were imported into China from the Maluku Islands. Chinese courtiers would pop a clove in their mouth to keep bad breath away whenever in the august presence of the almighty Chinese emperor.

Trade from Maluku to the Red and Mediterranean Sea ports of Ancient Greece, Egypt, and Rome was conducted via the ports of India's east coast. Boats would make it to the Malacca straits crossing to reach the Indian East Coast seaboard. They would then hug the coastline and make their journey down to the ports of the Southern Indian Peninsula before reaching Sri Lanka. Going around Cape Comorin, they would touch the Western coastline of India. The journey along the Western Indian seaboard would bring them to the Persian Gulf. Ports dotted the whole of this coastline from India to the Persian Gulf.

Goods intended for destinations beyond Mesopotamia could either continue this sea route crossing the Persian Gulf to follow the coastline of the Arabian Peninsula and enter the Red Sea. Others would take the land route after landing at the Mesopotamian ports to cross Syria and reach the Red Sea.

Trade caravans for the Red Sea region would also start from the ports of Oman and Yemen. They crossed the Arabian Desert in early first millennia BC on donkey caravans. Once camels were domesticated, camel caravans became the norm. Silk Road was the popular trade route to bring goods from China into West Asia and beyond.

Confucius (551-479 BC), in his Analects, mentions the use of ginger in food. In the 5th century AD, Chinese ships carried ginger plants onboard. Ginger gave freshness to food. They also believed that by eating ginger, scurvy could be prevented, a notion which modern science has proved to be false. Scurvy is caused from the deficiency of vitamin C, and ginger is not a source of this vitamin. Ginger, however, did help mask the staleness of food kept onboard—

probably the main reason for keeping ginger plants on ships undertaking transcontinental journeys.

Chinese food is not as spicy as Indian food. China is a vast country, and the food varies from region to region. Sichuan food is hot and rich in ginger and garlic, whereas the food in other places is mild.

The most popular Chinese herbs used in cooking are cassia, aloe vera, cloves, tea, alfafa, and ginger. These plants were preferred not just for their taste but also for their medicinal properties. An indicator of the importance given to herbs is the fact that one of the provinces in China is named after cassia[1] (Kwelin, which goes by the local name "kwei").

India

Northwestern India, including those regions that today form part of Pakistan and Afghanistan, Persia, Central Asia, Greece, and Rome, was a region of intense political and economic interaction from the 6th century BC to 5thcentury AD. This interaction was largely in the form of trade, business, knowledge, and cultural and religious exchange.

The word "globalization" is most commonly associated with the world of the 21st century but would also be relevant to this period. Persian and European kings from Cyrus the Great (538-530 BC), Darius I (521-486 BC), and Alexander the Great (born c. 325 BC), actively interacted with the kingdoms ruling northern and southern parts of the Indian subcontinent.

Megasthenes (350-290 BC) and many other Greek philosophers have recorded their impressions of India. The original writing of Megasthenes is, unfortunately, lost. But much of what he said comes to us from the Greeks who came to India after him. (Megasthenes was the Greek Ambassador to the court of the Mauryan Emperor Chandragupta. He wrote a book on his India experience, Indica.)

Asian Herbs

1   Cassia tastes almost identical to cinnamon. It is often sold as cinnamon. Details on the two spices can be read in Holy Herbs by Sudhir Ahluwalia (2017).

There existed between Greek dominions and India an active trade in incense, spices, textiles, silk, metals, glassware, slaves, etc. India was a major producer of spices and herbs. Megasthenes, Arrian,[2] and Pliny the Elder[3] have all, in their writings, named many Indian ports which traded with Greece and Rome. From these, Muziris appears to be a chief port of the Indian West Coast, lying close to the modern Kochi port in South India.

Pliny the Elder makes a mention of Kingdom of Pandya too. Pandyas are said to have ruled from 6th century to the 17th century AD although these dates are debated. Their dominions cover the region that corresponds to the modern state of Tamil Nadu in South India. Strabo (64 BC - 23 AD) mentions that the Pandyan King maintained diplomatic relations with Augustus Caesar. Pandyan ports were used to export spices and other goods to Rome, Greece, and the Red Sea and Persian Gulf regions.

The Red Sea region was under the political control of Imperial Rome during this period. Ships would cover the distance between the Red Sea and India in just ten days on the back of the southwest monsoon winds. Records from the Mauryan times (322-185 BC) show that, in addition to commonly traded spices like long pepper, cumin, coriander, cloves, turmeric, mustard, etc., there existed an active trade in numerous forms of salt including rock, sea, bida, and nitre.

2   Arrian was a Greek historian and philosopher who lived in the Roman period. He is best known for his book on the campaigns of Alexander – Anabasis of Alexander. He is said to have lived from 86/89 AD to 146/160 AD (https://en.wikipedia.org/wiki/Arrian).

3   Gaius Plinus Secundus, better known as Pliny the Elder, was a Roman author and naturalist and natural history philosopher of the early Roman period. He lived from 23 AD to 79 AD and is credited with writing the encyclopedic work Naturalis Historia (https:// en.wikipedia.org/wiki/Pliny_the_Elder).

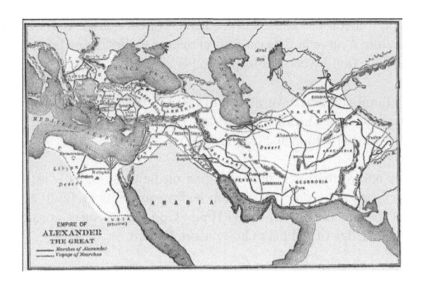

Picture 2: Empire of Alexander the Great

Source: A History of the Ancient World by George Willis Botsford Ph.D., published by The MacMillan Company in 1913.

Ayurveda literature has extensive references to herbs, plants, and spices. Sushrutasamhita and Charakasamhita are Ayurveda's two most prominent medical compilations. These works mention medicinal formulations made from imported and indigenous herbs. Herbs were also used as cosmetics.

Medical formulations were generally a combination of herbs, inorganic substances, and animal products. Treatment prescriptions include enunciation of chants and following prescribed rituals. The two were regarded to be integral to healing. Many of the medical formulations mentioned in these ancient compilations are still in use.

Siddha and Ayurveda

It is from palm leaf records in Tamil that we discover that there existed an herbal and mineral based ancient medicine system—Siddha. This system is different from Ayurveda. The earliest references to Siddha medicine are found in the ancient Tamil work Tholkappium.[4]

Ancient Tamil contained words from Prakrit, a language that was spoken in the northern state of Magadh (modern day Bihar state in East India). Literature on Siddha was written in ancient Tamil.

Siddha is one of the three ancient Indian medicine systems, with Ayurveda and Unani being the other two. Palm leaf manuscripts in Tamil ascribe the origin of the Siddha system to the Hindu God Shiva. Shiva is said to have passed knowledge of Siddha to his consort, Parvati.

Basic concepts of Siddha are like Ayurveda. Both claim that there exists an interrelationship between diet, lifestyle, and a healthy body and that herbs, minerals, exercise, and meditation together lead to healing.

Fundamentally, all ancient medical systems, including the ancient Greek and Egyptian systems, lay emphasis on nutrition and physical and mental exercise to keep the body free of ailments. Herbs and minerals were prescribed to support healing, but emphasis was on the former.

If this does not prove effective, combinations of herbs, minerals, and animal products are advised. According to the Siddha system, there exist in nature five elements: earth, water, fire, air, and ether. Together, these constitute all living beings.

There exists an intimate connection between the external world and the human body. Element of Earth is present in the bone, flesh, nerves, skin, and hair. Water is present in bile, blood, semen, glandular secretions, and sweat. Fire is part of hunger, thirst, sleep, beauty, and indolence.

---

4   Tholkappium is dated to the Sangam period that existed from around 300 BC to 300 AD. Scholars dispute these dates. Legend has it that there were three Sangam periods of

which the first two are wrapped in mythology.

Air enables contraction, expansion, and motion. Ether is present in the interstices of the stomach, heart, neck, and head. Effective medication is the interplay of these elements. Herbs and minerals help restore imbalances.

Yoga and Ayurveda, on the other hand, were based on Vedic thinking. Yoga defines human lifestyle. It includes exercise, meditation, and lifestyle practices. Ayurveda literally means "knowledge of life" and is an upaveda—an auxiliary of knowledge to Atharva Veda.

Atharva Veda is one of the four Vedas that form the basis of Vedic thinking. The Vedas are core to Hindu thinking. Atharva Veda contains hymns and incantations which help cure disease. Dhanvantari, the Hindu God of medicine, is believed to have received the knowledge of Ayurveda[5] from Brahma, one of the three gods that form the Hindu religion's trinity.

Four forms of remedies are mentioned in the Vedas. These are:

1.Atharvavani, which comes from Atharva Veda
2.Aangirasi, which is attributed to a mythological rishi or saint named Angirasa
3.Daivi or Divine
4.Majushayaja or beneficial to the common people

---

5   Ayurveda is divided into eight branches. These are:
1.Kaaya Chikitsa (Internal Medicine),
2.Baala Chikitsa (Treatment of Children/Pediatrics),
3.Graha Chikitsa (Demonology/Psychology),
4.Urdhvaanga Chikitsa (Treatment of disease above the clavicle),
5.Shalya Chikitsa (Surgery),
6.Damstra Chikitsa (Toxicology),
7.Jara Chikitsa (Geriatrics, Rejuvenation), and
8.Vrsha Chikitsa (Aphrodisiac therapy).

There are two major scholars who have been responsible for consolidating the knowledge of Ayurveda—Sushruta and Charaka.

Sushrutasamhita was penned in the 6th century BC, and in its extant form, has 184 chapters with descriptions of 1,120 illnesses, 700 medicinal plants, 64 preparations from mineral sources, and 57 preparations based on animal sources. This work is largely focused on surgery. Charakasamhita focuses on internal medicine and was penned by Charaka who probably lived in the 4th century BC.

According to the Foundation for Revitalization of Local Health Traditions, India ("FRLHT," an organization specializing in Indian medicinal plants), Charakasamhita has 1,990 plants and its variants listed therein. Of these, research has been conducted on 650 plants. Over 500 Ayurvedic drugs have been prepared for commercial use from the plants listed in Charakasamhita.

These compilations are of immense value as they constitute a break from the ancient Vedic tradition where knowledge was passed from one generation to the other orally. The two samhitas were subsequently translated into Arabic by Muslim scholars, and later, into English. Other notable works on Ayurveda include the Madhava Nidham (7th century AD), Shrangadharasamhita (15thcentury AD), and Bhava Prakasha (16th century AD).

Unani System

The connection of India with the Mediterranean and Middle Eastern regions was further strengthened by the introduction of Unani medicine by the Arabs in India in the 12th century AD. Unani has its origin in the Middle East. It developed into a full-fledged medical system under Arabic and Persian physicians including Rhazes (850-925 AD), Avicenna (980-1037 AD), and Al Zahrawi (936-1013 AD), among others.

Avicenna wrote his now famous work, The Canon of Medicine, in Persia, circa 1025 AD, based on the teachings of Hippocrates (c. 460-377 BC) and

Galen (131-210 AD). When Persia and the Muslim world was conquered by the Mongols in the 12th century AD, large numbers of scholars of Unani medicine fled to India. In India, the system grew and flourished under the patronage of the Delhi Sultanate, and later Mughal rulers. Upon reaching the subcontinent, the system was influenced by Ayurvedic practices. Today, Unani medicine is very similar to Ayurveda.

According to Unani medicine, the key elements impacting the human body are air, earth, water, and fire, an imbalance in which causes disease. Treatments, which often include various herbal combinations, are aimed at rebalancing these elements. As was common to all ancient medicinal systems, the focus in Unani too is on diet and digestion.

There are six essential prerequisites in the prevention of diseases—air, food and drink, bodily and physical movement, repose, sleep and wakefulness, retention, and evacuation.

In post-independence India, the Unani system received continued government support. A survey of medicinal plants across India has been conducted by the government and an herbarium of plants created. Despite this support, Unani's share in the current market for alternate medicine is just 2.3% which is put at $1 billion in the United States. In another blow, Unani medicine is not a recognized or licensed health profession in North America.

CHAPTER II

Globally used Aromatic Plants from India

Incense emanating cisterns recovered during excavations of the cities of the Indus Valley indicate the use of incense. It was a Bronze Age civilization with substantial capability in logistics management. Copper was imported to the Indus Valley cities from distant areas in Central India and precious stones from Western and Northern Afghanistan. An active trade via the sea thrived with the Mesopotamian (the area which is modern day Iraq) Civilization. It cultivated crops like wheat, barley, lentils, peas, cotton, and sesame and reared animals like humped cattle, goats, and sheep.

Archaeological excavations have unearthed figurines of women wearing pearls, fillets, brooches, hairpins, ear and nose ornaments, armlets, bracelets, bangles, finger rings, and girdles. Sticks of kohl, still used to shade the eyes, have also been found from the Indus Valley sites. Interestingly, even after two millennia, we can see continued use of similar jewelry by people in India.

Unlike the Mesopotamian ancient Egyptian civilizations where tablets and papyrus writings have supplemented archaeological findings, only seals with inscriptions have been recovered from the Indus Valley Civilization areas. Seals do show some markings, but whether this is evidence of the existence of a script used by the Indus Valley Civilization is a question that is yet to be answered. Shereen Ratnagar opines that these seals were probably used to designate ownership of a property (Ratnagar, 2001).

Archaeological evidence, and analysis of preserved food elements in pots, has revealed the use of traditional spices, herbs, cosmetics, and incenses. These spices and herbs continue to be used in India.

The next major civilization in the subcontinent of South Asia began with the Vedic period. The Vedic age in South Asia is said to have begun c. 1750 BC in the dying throes of the Indus Valley Civilization. The Indo-Aryans, as these people were called, perhaps migrated from the Central Asian region bordering modern-day China and Russia. This theory is disputed by scholars who opine that the Aryan people in were indigenous to South Asia.

Other scholars opine that the Indo-Aryans, over time, were divided into two branches—one that migrated and occupied territories of modern-day Iran, Iraq, Syria, and maybe some parts of Turkey, and the other that moved eastwards into Afghanistan, Pakistan, and Northern India. With time, these people moved southwards into the Deccan Plateau.

The Indus Valley population got displaced by these aggressive migrants forcing the indigenous residents to move south and occupy southern parts of India. The Aryans are credited for enunciating the Vedas. The Vedas codify the beliefs, practices, and thinking of these people, and form the foundation of Hindu religious thinking. Vedic knowledge is enshrined in the four Vedas—Rigveda, Yajurveda, Samaveda, and Atharvaveda.

In addition to the Vedas were the six Vedangas. The Vedangas identified are Siksha, Nirukta, Chhanda, Vyakarna, Jyotisha, and Kalpa. There were other supportive texts created by the Vedic people; they include Meemamsa which are interpretations, Nyaya (logic), Puranas, and Shastras.

The Indo-Aryans were a tribal and pastoral society who eventually settled down into an agricultural community. They had always been closely associated with nature, and their gods, food, herbs, spices, and medicine all came from nature. This intimate connection with nature, herbs, and plants is exemplified in the hymn, an ode to herbs, quoted below from the oldest of the Vedas, Rigveda.

Praise of Herbs

HERBS that sprang up in time of old, three ages earlier than the Gods—

Of these, whose hue is brown, will I declare the hundred powers and seven.
 Ye, Mothers, have a hundred homes, yea, and a thousand are your growths.

Do ye who have a thousand powers free this my patient from disease.
Be glad and joyful in the Plants, both blossoming and bearing fruit,
Plants that will lead us to success like mares who conquer in the race.

Plants, by this name I speak to you, Mothers, to you the Goddesses:
Steed, cow, and garment may I win, win back thy very self, O man. The
Holy Fig tree is your home, your mansion is the Parna tree:

Winners of cattle shall ye be if ye regain for me this man.

He who hath store of Herbs at hand like Kings amid a crowd of men—

Physician is that sage's name, fiend-slayer, chaser of disease.

Herbs rich in Soma, rich in steeds, in nourishments, in strengthening power—

All these have I provided here, that this man may be whole again. The
healing virtues of the Plants stream forth like cattle from the stall—

Plants that shall win me store of wealth, and save thy vital breath, O man.

Reliever is your mother's name, and hence Restorers are ye called.

Sudhir Ahluwalia

Rivers are ye with wings that fly: keep far whatever brings disease.

Over all fences have they passed, as steals a thief into the fold.

The Plants have driven from the frame whatever malady was there. When, bringing back the vanished strength, I hold these herbs within my hand,

The spirit of disease departs ere he can seize upon the life.

He through whose frame, O Plants, ye creep member by member, joint by joint—

From him ye drive away disease like some strong arbiter of strife.

Fly, Spirit of Disease, begone, with the blue jay and kingfisher.

Fly with the wind's impetuous speed, vanish together with the storm. Help every one the other, lend assistance each of you to each,

All of you be accordant, give furtherance to this speech of mine. Let fruitful Plants, and fruitless, those that blossom, and the blossomless,

Urged onward by Bṛhaspati, release us from our pain and grief; Release me from the curse's plague and woe that comes from Varuṇa; Free me from Yama's fetter, from sin and offence against the Gods. What time, descending from the sky, the Plants flew earthward, thus they spake:

No evil shall befall the man whom while he liveth we pervade,

Of all the many Plants whose King is, Soma, Plants of hundred forms, Thou art the Plant most excellent, prompt to the wish, sweet to the heart.

O all ye various Herbs whose King is Soma, that o'erspread the earth,

Urged onward by Bṛhaspati, combine your virtue in this Plant. Unharmed be he who digs you up, unharmed the man for whom I dig:

And let no malady attack biped or quadruped of ours.

All Plants that hear this speech, and those that have departed far away,

Come all assembled and confer your healing power upon this Herb. With Soma as their Sovran Lord the Plants hold colloquy and say: O King, we save from death the man whose cure a Brahman undertakes. Most excellent of all art thou, O Plant thy vassals are the trees.

Let him be subject to our power, the man who seeks to injure us. (Rigveda translation by Ralph. TH. Griffith, 1896)

This hymn, like many other references to plants in other literary and secular literature, is evidence of the importance of nature in ancient human society. I see commonalities in thought between the Vedic hymns and the Biblical verses that praise and stress the importance of plants, herbs, and spices. I was particularly impressed by the following verse in the Bible, a lesson in conservation which is relevant to the world now more than ever before:

Deuteronomy 20:19

"When you besiege a city a long time, to make war against it in order to capture it, you shall not destroy its trees by swinging an axe against them; for you may eat from them, and you shall not cut them down. For is the tree of the field a man, that it should be besieged by you?"

Trees and plants were valued by humans across cultures, religions, and civilizations. The importance given to the planting of trees is illustrated by the following hadith:

"If a Muslim plants a tree or sows seeds, and then a bird, or a person or an animal eats from it, it is regarded as a charitable gift (sadaqah) for

him."
-Imam Bukhari (Sahih al Bukhari 2320, Book 41, Hadith 1, Vol 3, Book 39, Hadith 513)

Greek and Indian medicinal thought both lay great stress on lifestyle. Treatment is based on an individual's constitution. In India, the focus was, and to some extent still is, on Yogic exercises, and physical and spiritual lifestyle. These assist healing and promote well-being.

While there are many differences between the Greek and India societies, one of the commonalities is the intimate connection of the two with nature. Ancient Greek, Vedic, and even Egyptian gods were based in nature.

The Vedic period in India began around the period between 1500 BC and 1750 BC. Gods were propitiated with yajna (sacred fire) accompanied by rituals, including animal sacrifices. Verses from the Vedas were recited as aromatic herbs and spices were added to yajna fire.
The fragrance emanating from herbs added to the holy fire helped create a pleasant ambience. Some of these practices have endured time. Aromatic herbs continue to be added to yajnafires in modern India, though animal sacrifices have largely disappeared. However, buffalo sacrifice before the Hindu goddess of death, Kali, still exists in Eastern India.

In Ancient Egyptian and Greek medicine, as well as in Ayurveda, aroma from herbs and chants of hymns were integral to healing practices, elevating the mood and calming the mind. Incense and spices also helped purify the air. These form the basis of modern aromatherapy too.

Offerings or oblations of aromatic and medicinal herbs, resins, barks, leaves, exudates (gums which flow from trees), twigs, roots, and seeds, along with foodstuffs and ghee (clarified butter) were made to the sacred fires. The offerings were made to Agni, the god of fire who, according to mythology, carried them to the celestial world.

Yajnas were performed on almost all-important occasions—weddings, births, deaths, coronations, and in praise and appeasement of the gods. The most common plants used as incense in yajnas are sandalwood, basil, cedar wood, cassia, vetiver, turmeric, and cloves, among others. The traditional well-known scents of ancient India were jasmine, rose, sandalwood, champa, cedar and musk, all of which originate from plants or animals found in the region.

Ancient Sanskrit literature has references to the use of incense in homes and in streets during festivities. On joyous occasions, fragrant water was sprayed on streets and thoroughfares; scented flower garlands would adorn and decorate entranceways of homes. Even today, during the Hindu Festival of Light, Diwali, and other festivals, it is common for people to decorate their homes with leaves from the mango tree and garlands made from marigold and jasmine flowers.

Flowers and herbs have deep spiritual connotations in Hindu philosophy. They were and continue to be the chief sources of incense in India. Incense sticks and dhoop (made from the aromatic sap of a tree or shrub) are a part of the 16 essential offerings in a typical Hindu ritual— the others being betel leaf, betel nut, camphor, cardamom, cloth, clove, diya (lamp), grain, naivedhyam (a mix of nine offerings), sandalwood paste, sweets, and water.

In Ayurveda, biological energies that are found in the body and mind are called the doshas. They are said to govern the living being and derive their properties from the five elements described in the Vedas, i.e., earth, water, fire, space, and air. The three doshas identified in Ayurveda are Vata which is composed of space and air, Pitta of fire and water, and Kapha of earth and water.

There is a deep and intimate connection between aroma and good health in Ayurveda. Aromas are said to increase or decrease the human body's ether/air (Vata), fire/oil (Pitta), and water/earth (Kapha) compositions. Aromas can be important additions to living a harmonious Ayurvedic lifestyle.

Aromas are classified since their impact on the body. For example, sweet aromas like that of sandalwood possess a cooling property, while musk is pungent and stimulating with aphrodisiac qualities. It is excellent for cultivating bhakti or devotional links with deities. For illustration, some examples of beneficial incenses and oils for each of the three humors of Ayurveda are given below:

Vata: Musk, sandalwood, and rose.
Pitta: Sandalwood, rose, and lavender.
Kapha: Cedar, myrrh, and musk.

SANDALWOOD (Santalum album)- Incense that helps you relax

This is a mid-sized evergreen tree that is usually 4-9 meters in height. There are three major species of sandalwood: Santalum album, Santalum spicatum, and Santalum lanceolatum. Santalum album is native to a wide ecology from the semi-evergreen to dry deciduous tropical forests of Southern India. This tree is the source of the popular sandalwood oil.

S. spicatum and S. lanceolatum are two other commercially valuable sources of sandalwood oil and are found in Australia. S. spicatum is the more popular and important of the two and is widely grown in Western Australia. The significant difference between the Australian and the Indian sandalwood varieties is that the latter has much higher levels of santalol[6] (60-70 percent as compared to 25-30 percent in Australian species).

High levels of santalol give a very high-top note[7] to Indian sandalwood. It is the top note that you smell first. The base note is important in aromatherapy and is the same for both species.

---

6   Santalol is an organic compound—sesquiterpene. It is responsible for the sweet aroma of sandalwood. There are two variants of santalol (alpha and beta santalol) that are found in sandalwood trees.
7   Top note is described as "the dominant initial element of a fragrance that dissipates quickly."

Sandalwood oil from S. spicatum is used as a fixative. The Australian species oil is more resinous, drier, and has a less sweet note. Sandalwood oil from Australia is mainly exported to China.

Although the trees in the wild can live up to one hundred years, the age at which it can be commercially exploited, for either the fragrant wood or sandalwood oil, is forty years. The demand for the wood and oil is much more than the supply available. S. album has become highly

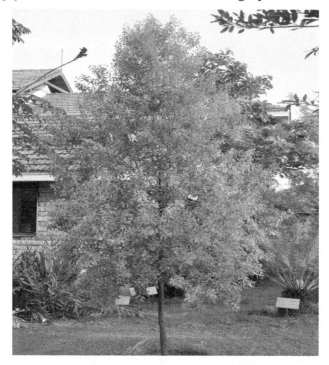

Picture 3: Santalum album
Photo By: Dr Ravikumar, Senior Botanist FRLHT

depleted due to overexploitation. To protect the species, the Indian government has nationalized it. Logging and extraction of sandalwood trees are prohibited, except by the state.

A thriving black market for smuggled sandalwood exists in India. Trees that have attained exploitable diameter are frequently targeted by smugglers and illegal loggers. To protect sandalwood trees, all trees growing on private land must be enumerated and a declaration made before the local forestry official. Any theft of sandalwood is to be immediately reported to the forest authorities.

Despite these precautions and controls, smugglers resort to illegal logging of sandalwood trees both in the wild and on private land. Smugglers enter forests in the dead of night, strip the bark, and remove the sapwood which is low in fragrant oil content, exposing the oil-rich heartwood. This is cut into small billets and stowed in bags and transported.

Efforts to cultivate sandalwood in plantations in India to supplement the stock available in the wild have achieved mixed results. I have seen successful plantations of Santalum album in the Mysore region of Karnataka state, India. Privately owned plantations have also been raised in the neighboring Tamil Nadu.

Sandalwood seedlings are raised in nurseries from a host plant that is seeded with the sandalwood seed. The tree is a hemi-parasite as it is dependent, in the initial stages of its life, on the host's roots. The haustoria of Santalum penetrate and draw nourishment from the root of the host plant. The tree soon becomes independent and able to thrive without the host.

There is sustained demand for sandalwood. Sandalwood is hard and close grained with a very hard aromatic heartwood. Termites find it difficult to eat through the wood. The wood is prized by artisans who carve intricate figures and designs on the wood, especially in South India where the craftsmanship is exemplary.

Master craftsmen spend an entire lifetime making intricate carvings on sandalwood. Traditionally, craftsmen have focused their artistry on carving figures of Hindu gods, goddesses, and animals, mainly elephants. Non-religious designs wereundertaken against specific orders. These carvings are coveted not only for their intricate design but also for the fragrance of the wood.

A mature tree, aged around 40 to 50 years, can yield up to 250 kilograms of sandalwood oil. The heartwood contains around 2-5% oil, but the roots yield more (6-7%). Sandalwood oil has a sweet and woody fragrance.

Most sandalwood produced in India is used by the local soap and cosmetic industries. Exports are mainly to the US and the Middle East. There, it is used in manufacturing of sandal-scented cosmetic creams, lotions, soaps, perfumes, and skincare products. The fragrance of the oil is mild and long lasting. Sandalwood perfume blends well with other perfumes.

Historical Overview and Use in Religion

The oldest recorded mention of sandalwood goes back to the 5th century BC. References to the wood have been traced to a Nirukta, or commentary on the Vedas. There is evidence of sandalwood use in Ancient Egypt too, where the oil was used as fragrance and to perfume the mummies of the Pharaohs. Sandalwood was also used as incense in Ancient Egyptian temples as the scent was believed to drive out evil spirits.

In Hinduism, the wood was dedicated to the god Shiva and was used in temples both as timber for construction and to make statues of the gods. According to the Hindu faith, sandalwood aids in achieving higher levels of reincarnation. [8] Deceased Hindu rulers were embalmed with the essential oil or with sandalwood paste. Even today, funeral pyre of the rich and powerful Indians is built with sandalwood. India's first Prime Minister, Jawaharlal Nehru, was cremated on a funeral pyre of sandalwood, as were those of the princes killed in the epic battle of Mahabharata. Scholars place the Mahabharata[9] at around the 8th or 9th century BC.

---

8 The Hindus believe that every living being has a soul which, on its demise, enters another living body. This process of re-birth is called reincarnation. A human body is believed to be acquired by a soul after multiple levels of reincarnation from the lowest animal forms to the highest – that of a human.
9   The Mahabharata was an ancient tribal war fought on the plains of Haryana state near Kurukshetra in Northern India.

Mahabharata is one of the two most revered ancient Hindu epics. Buddhist, the Pandava king was shown arranging for sandalwood to cremate his mentor, Bhishma, the patriarch warrior, who had been killed in battle with Arjuna, his brother. The following verse explains this:

Pious rites are due to foemen and to friends and kinsmen slain, None shall lack a fitting funeral, none shall perish on the plain.

Wise Vidura and his comrades sped on sacred duty bound, Sandalwood and scented aloes, fragrant oil and perfumes found. (The Ramayana and the Mahabharata – Condensed into English Verse by Romesh C Dutt, 2012)

Burning of fragrant sandalwood twigs in sacred fires in Zoroastrian temples was a common practice. In Buddhism, sandalwood, aloes wood, and cloves were used as incense in temples. There are references to sandalwood in the Bible too:

1 Kings 10:12

> The king used the algumwood to make supports for the temple of the Lord and for the royal palace, and to make harps and lyres for the musicians.

There are references to use of sandalwood paste in Islamic Sufi sects. In yoga, sandalwood is linked to the Root Chakra, said to awaken the kundalini snake which leads to enhanced libido.

It is also used in Shinto shrines in Japan. A piece of sandalwood is rubbed against a piece of granite, and a paste is made with the wood dust and water. This paste is used to anoint foreheads, necks, and chests of Hindu deities, priests, and worshippers. Sandalwood paste is also used in many Hindu and Buddhist religious ceremonies.

Arab physicians brought sandalwood to Europe in the Middle Ages, where it first appeared in Italian pharmacies during the 15th century.

In Perfumes and Skin Care

Sandalwood is used in perfume compositions, especially the Indian attars (local perfumes). Sandalwood oil is used to create perfume blends as it blends well with most oils like clove bud, lavender, geranium, patchouli, jasmine, benzoin, bergamot, clary sage, coriander, cypress,
  fennel, frankincense, galbanum, myrrh, palmarosa, pepper black, and peppermint.

Sandalwood has a rich, balsamic, sweet fragrance with delicate wood notes, and a bright and fresh edge with few natural analogues. The fragrance of sandalwood has relaxing properties, reduces stress, and promotes restful sleep. It is reputed to be an aphrodisiac. When used in smaller proportions in a perfume, it is an excellent fixative and enhances other fragrances.

The color of the oil is between pale yellow and pale gold. It is widely used in the cosmetic industry, given its value as a skincare product. It provides relief to dry, cracked, and chapped skin, rashes, and acne. It is suitable for all skin types and is non-toxic. The oil relieves itching and inflammation of the skin and is most effective on dehydrated skin. It is well regarded for its anti-aging skincare properties. The astringent action has a great toning effect.

The oil is said to be effective in getting rid of skin scars and is used to fight dry eczema. It is a key ingredient in many Ayurvedic skin care treatments. Sandalwood powder can be ground into a paste, lotion, or used in soapmaking for its cleansing and hydrating properties. Sawdust from the heartwood is used as incense and in imparting fragrance to clothes and cupboards.

Almost all the sandalwood oil traded internationally is the so-called "East Indian" sandalwood oil which is distilled from the heartwood and roots of Santalum album. India and Indonesia are the two major producers and exporters of sandalwood oil, but reliable production data is not available.

The United States and France are the two largest importers of Indian sandalwood oil, along with the Middle East. The United States is the biggest market for sandalwood oil outside of India. Indian exports have averaged about 40 metric tons per annum. Indonesia is the only other supplier of the East Indian-type of sandalwood oil. Recorded annual exports over the six-year period of 1987-1992 averaged 15 metric tons.

Indian sandalwood oil has up to 90% santalol content whereas the Australian variety has only 38-39%. The harvesting age of sandalwood trees in the wild is 40 years, but trees in plantations can be harvested at the age of 15 years as the formation of the heartwood in these trees starts early at just four to five years of age. Indian sandalwood oil contains 50-60% of alpha santalol and 15-25% of beta santalol.

In Medicine

When used externally, the oil and paste of sandalwood has a calming and cooling effect. Conditions like depression, anxiety, and insomnia can be eased with sandalwood aromatherapy as it is said to help relax the mind.

In Tibetan medicine, it is used in combination with other aromatics as a massage oil and incense. The oil is used to provide relief in cases of insomnia, anxiety, depression, nervous tension, stress-related conditions, and other psychological ailments. The sandalwood's smell helps induce restful sleep.

It is said to stimulate the immune system and is regarded as a good antiseptic. It is traditionally believed to assist in improving conditions of frigidity and impotence, and was used not just as perfume, but also as a natural aphrodisiac.

Sesquiterpenes, sesquiterpenols, sesquiterpenals, santalic and teresantalic acid, aldehyde, pterocarpin and hydrocarbons, isovaleric aldehyde, santene, and santenone are the molecules that have been isolated from sandalwood. Sandalwood oil was found to have anticarcinogenic, antiviral, and bactericidal activity. The anti-cancer effect of alpha santalol on prostate cancer was observed by Bommareddy, et al. in 2007.

The anti-cancer property of sandalwood oil and alpha santalol was also observed in studies conducted on animals (Santha et al., 2015).

Only the occasional case of skin irritation has been observed when sandalwood product is direct applied on the skin (Burdock et al., 2008).

An in-vitro study has shown that sandalwood oil is effective against methicillin-resistant Staphylococcus aureus (MRSA) and antimycotic-resistant Candida species In another study, a crude extract as well as isolated compounds of sandalwood oil (primarily α- and β-santalol)
 showed antibacterial activity against Helicobacter pylori, a Gram-negative bacterium which cause duodenal, gastric, and stomach ulcers (Ochi et al., 2005).

Sandalwood oil exhibited virulence against isolates of drug-resistant herpes simplex virus type I (Schnitzler et al., 2007). The anti-ulcer property of the hydro-alcoholic extracts of the stem of Santalum album was tested on wistar rats with positive results (Ahmed et al., 2013). Another study reports that β-santalol exhibited anti-influenza A/ HK (H3N2) virus activity (Paulpandi et al., 2012).

Sandalwood oil elevates pulse rate, the level of skin conductance and systolic blood pressure, and brings about increased attentiveness, uplifting the mood in humans (Heubeger et al., 2006).

CAMPHOR- the natural decongestant

Camphor, a highly flammable crystalline substance, has been in use in India since early Vedic times (c. 1750 BC). It was used to start the yajna fire lit to perform Vedic rituals and continues to be in use for Hindu rituals to this day.

Ancient Aryans are believed to have indulged in animal sacrifice. These offerings were made to Agni, the fire god. The aroma from the camphor and spices helped mask the foul smell of burning flesh, and their antiseptic property helped keep flies and insects away. Camphor is still used by Hindus to ignite a cremation pyre.

Ancient Jews, too, sacrificed animals at the Jewish temple. Holy anointing oil and incense was extensively used in the Jewish temple. The scents from these incenses helped mask the foul smell of burning sacrificial carcasses.

Camphor, in ancient times, was also used in embalming the dead by the Sumerians, Babylonians, Jews, Zoroastrians, and Egyptians. Products like camphor, which were used in the production of aromatic incenses, were imported into the region from Asia and Africa for such purposes.

About trade in camphor and other commodities, The Periplus of the Erythrean Sea wrote in a commentary around the 1st century AD:

> "We have been told through Indian as well as foreign literary sources that in ancient times, commodities like sugar, palm oil, coconut oil, cotton cloth, clarified butter, cast iron, tin sheets, copper vessels, dyes and pigments like cinnabar (ochre), indigo and lac, perfumes like sandalwood oil, musk tamarind, costs, maker, camphor, and even crude glass crockery were being exported from India."

(The Periplus of the Erythrina Sea – Travels and Trade in the Indian Ocean by a Merchant in the First Century, translated from the Greek and Annotated by Wilfred H. Schoff, Longmans Green and Co. New York, 1912)

References to camphor are found in the Bible and the Hadiths. Camphor is mentioned in writings attributed to the time of Prophet Mohammed:

> Prophet's daughter, Fāṭema, concerning the right amount of camphor for each ḥonūṭ: "When the Messenger of Allāh was on his deathbed, Gabriel brought him from Paradise forty dirhams of camphor, which he [the Prophet] divided into three portions: one-third for his own [ḥonūṭ], one-third for ʿAlī, and one-third for me."

(Encyclopedia Iranica)

It is widely accepted by scholars and historians that Arabs introduced natural camphor to Europe. There it was used as incense and in medicine. The use of natural camphor ended soon after the discovery of cheaper chemical alternatives.

Some translations wrongly equate henna with camphor. Henna comes from a bush growing in dry deciduous habitats of South Asia and the Middle East. Camphor, on the other hand, is extracted from camphor trees that inhabit moist, tropical, deciduous, semi-evergreen, and evergreen ecosystems.

Botany and Distribution

Camphor is obtained from two different genera and species of trees: Cinnamomum camphora, native to the tropical and sub-tropical evergreen ecosystems of China and Japan, and Dryobalanops camphora,

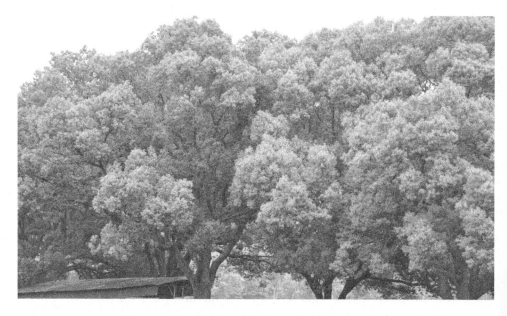

Picture 4: Cinnamomum camphora avenue
Photo: Dr Ravikumar, Senior Botanist FRLHT

native to Borneo. The aroma and properties of camphor obtained from these two species is similar.

Camphor trees are giant trees, growing up to forty meters in height. The leaves of this tree are glossy with a waxy texture, and are known for their ornamental, aromatic, and medicinal properties. The leaves and bark of the tree, when crushed, emit the scent that is commonly associated with camphor or Eucalyptus.

In the 1800s, camphor trees were introduced in habitats outside its natural zone, in Southeastern US, Hawaii, and Australia. In Australia, the plant was originally introduced as an ornamental shade tree and for the extraction of the then-popular camphor oil. Commercial use of the species, though, was never undertaken.

In Australia, the trees are called camphor laurels. (The commonly used word, laurel, is derived from the family Lauraceae to which the species belongs.) Today, the plant is regarded as an invasive pest, and planting and distribution of this tree is prohibited in New South Wales and Queensland.

The leaves from the trees clog waterways, disrupting drainage and irrigation. Camphor trees are observed to invade old pasturelands, a common feature of most exotic species. In an exotic ecosystem, the plant faces little competition from pests and diseases and finds it easy to oust native flora.

In Southeast US, particularly, in North and Central Florida, the species has become an invasive weed. It has been observed growing aggressively along the side of the roads, on fallow pastures, and on disturbed sites. Similar is the case in Hawaii where the exotic is now a major threat to the island's native flora.

Camphor is extracted from trees that have reached an age of fifty years or more. Camphor oil is extracted from the wood, root stumps, and branches. A single tree can yield up to three tons of camphor in both oil and solid form.

Wood chips contain approximately 5% of the essence of camphor (Janick, 1969).

Extraction is done by vacuum after wood chips are fed into an oil steam distillation still. To remove impurities from the oil, it is strained through a filter press, and three fractions of oil are produced—as white, yellow, and brown camphor. Only the white camphor oil fraction is put to commercial use. This fraction has a clear and fresh aroma.

The brown and yellow camphor fractions are toxic as they contain safrole, a carcinogenic molecule. Safrole is also found in other spices like nutmeg and pepper, but in a much smaller quantity. Camphor was earlier used as food flavor, but with the discovery of its carcinogenic properties, its use in food has been prohibited in the US by the FDA (Food and Drug Administration).

The camphor tree is cut, and its wood is converted into chips to extract the oil. Logging in evergreen and semi-evergreen ecosystems is ecologically destructive. A felled tree, when it falls onto the forest floor, damages the multi-storeyed flora of these ecosystems and also leaves a huge gap in the forest canopy. The soil in these gaps is exposed to erosion during heavy downpours, common in such areas. I have observed that in evergreen forests, even after selected felling (removal of single selected trees like for extracting camphor), the flora in the gaps take a very long time to recover.

Before alternative sources to camphor were discovered, heavy demand led to the overexploitation of camphor trees in nature, causing a rapid fall in the population of the species. In places like Taiwan, the species came close to extinction.

In Ancient Egypt and the surrounding region, camphor was used during embalming. The process of embalming starts with disemboweling the body and drying it with salt. The body is then wrapped in linen soaked in resins from fir, pine trees, beeswax, myrrh, palm wine, cassia, camphor oil, etc., for preservation. All these herbs have drying and antibacterial properties.

Potteryware dated as far back as 3150 BC was subjected to chemical analysis. The results reveal that resins and oils including camphor was used to flavor ancient wines (Mc Govern et al., 2008).

As Medicine

Camphor was used to fumigate localities affected by plague, outbreaks of which were common in the ancient world, including Egypt (Chen et al., 2013). In Persia, too, it was a viewed as a remedy against plague.

Camphor was used as perfume and medicine in Egypt in the first and second millennia, as noted in Ebers Papyrus (c. 1550 BC). They also used it to treat epilepsy. The strong aroma of camphor was used by Ancient Greeks to revive someone who had fainted.

Atharva Veda makes a mention of rubbing camphor on the abdomen as a treatment for urine retention. The treatment was accompanied by chants and mantras.

In Ayurveda, camphor mixed with oil is used to gain relief from inflammation caused by arthritis, sprains, rheumatism, and muscular pains. The oil acts on the sensory nerves of the peripheral nervous system and subdues the inflammation. A mix of camphor, Eucalyptus, and other oils is used for a synergistic effect.

Camphor has a dual hot -and-cold action. When first applied, the oil numbs the muscles and emanates a feeling of coolness. Slowly, this cooling is replaced by a warmth as the blood flow to the affected region increases, reducing the stress and leading to reduced inflammation.
A study on rats validates the anti-arthritic property of camphor (Li et al., 2009).

There is not enough evidence to support its use in treating toenail fungus, hemorrhoids, warts, etc., although it is prescribed for these ailments in

Ayurveda. Other Ayurvedic applications include use in cardiac stimulation, as a remedy for hysteria, and to treat diarrhea.

The historically celebrated medicinal properties of camphor are its anti-inflammatory, antiseptic, anti-microbial, anesthetic, anti-flatulent, stimulant, and pain-relieving characteristics. The oil was used to treat nervous depression, acne, inflammation, bronchitis, coughs, colds, fever, flu, etc.

Overdose can lead to convulsions and vomiting, especially in pregnant women. People suffering from epilepsy and asthma were advised against use of camphor. Camphor oil is no longer used in aromatherapy as it is suspected to be a convulsant and neurotoxin.

Camphor is used to decongest the chest, as an expectorant and a febrifuge. Several camphor-based decongestants are available in the market, like the popular Vicks VapoRub™.

Camphor's anti-inflammatory, antiviral, and antibacterial properties make it a popular remedy for cold, flu, and bronchitis. A study showed that the compound named cinnamaldehyde present in camphor helps retard the progression of adenovirus (the common cold virus responsible for upper respiratory tract ailments) (Liu et al., 2009).

It is a common practice to inhale camphor to reduce the urge to cough. However, this is an unsafe practice as the ingestion of camphor can cause serious side effects, even death.
Use of camphorated oils was banned in the US in the 1980s, though it is still in use in Canada and other parts of the world. With a rise in awareness of negative effects of camphor, use of camphor as medicine has decreased.

Camphor is also used topically as an eardrop, to treat minor burns, relieve pain, and reduce itching. It is commonly used in combination with menthol in over-the-counter cooling and anti-itch gels. These topical applications are still permitted in the US as only oral medicines were banned in the '80s, but the FDA has restricted total camphor content to 11%.

Current medical opinion accepts camphor's use in relieving a cough when applied as a chest rub, for treating itching and irritation of the skin (bruises, minor burns, insect bites, etc.), and to provide relief from pain.

Camphor should not be directly applied to broken skin as it enters the body rapidly and is poisonous in high concentrations. Camphor is a very toxic substance and numerous cases of camphor poisoning (Chen et al., 2013) have been documented.
Camphor contains a range of alkaloids and molecules like alpha pinene, camphene, b-pinene, limonene, cinnamaldehyde, eugenol, etc. These molecules have been isolated, identified, and tested by scientists. Two compounds, linalool and camphor, have been isolated from Cinnamomum camphora trees in Brazil (Frizzo et al., 2000).

The anti-fungal properties of the essential oil were validated in a study. (Pragadheesh et al., 2013). The anti-depressant properties that have traditionally been attributed to camphor oil were studied and validated through experiments on rats (Rabadia et al., 2013). Camphor oil was observed to reduce human sperm mobility, leading to the claim that the oil has contraceptive properties (Mansee et al., 2010).

Other Uses

In China and several other parts of the world where camphor trees are found in abundance, its wood was used in ship building. The leaves are widely used as a culinary spice and as an ingredient in products like incense, insect repellents, and flea killing pesticide. Moth balls were made from camphor until it was replaced by naphthalene.

It is also used as a remover on oil paint and varnish. Other uses include as a plasticizer in nitrocellulose, a material used in explosives. Solid camphor releases fumes which form a coating that protects against rusting. Therefore, storing tool kits with solid camphor will keep rust away.

Camphor can help remove excess oil from the skin and is used in the cosmetics industry. It is an ingredient in face washes, clarifying masks, and astringents. Camphor is also used as a flavoring agent in sweets, confectionary, and deserts in Asia and Arabia. Camphor oil blends particularly well with basil, cajuput, chamomile, lavender, etc.

HOLY BASIL – the miracle medicinal plant

Holy Basil or tulsi is an aromatic plant held in reverence by Hindus. The plant has been revered in India for thousands of years as it is regarded as the incarnation of Vishnu, one of the trinity of the Hindu Pantheon. The herb occupies a place of pride at the center of the courtyard in most Hindu homes. It is not uncommon for Hindus to keep a tulsi plant in a pot even in high-rise apartments these days, indicating the reverence it commands.

The plant is described by some as the "The Mother Medicine of Nature" and is referred to as such in ancient Hindu literature. An ode to the plant in the Kanva Sakha branch of the Vedas is quoted below:

Of all flowers, Tulsi is the best. She is worshipable and beautiful and burns up the fuel of sins like a flame of fire. Of all the goddesses, she is the most sacred. Because no one can compare to her, she is called Tulsi. I worship this goddess who is entreated by all. She is placed on the heads of all, desired by all, and makes the universe holy. She bestows liberation from this world and devotion to Lord Hari[10]. I worship her.

The plant is attributed to possess mythical properties in Hindu literature.

> "Every home with a Tulsi plant is a place of pilgrimage and no disease, messengers of Yama, the God of death can enter it."
> – Skandapurana, 2, 4, 8, 13 Padmapurana Uttarakhanda

---

10   Hari is synonymous to Hindu God Vishnu

There exist references to tulsi in the oldest of Vedic texts—the Rig Veda. The following extract from the Patalkanda
of the Padmapurana illustrates the worship of tulsi:

> One who hears Tulsi Devi's glories will have all his sinful reactions, stored from many births, destroyed and very quickly attain the lotus-feet of Sri Sri Radha-Krishna.

> The leaves, flowers, roots, bark, branches, trunk and the shade of Tulsi Devi are all spiritual.

One, whose dead body is burnt in a fire, which has Tulsi wood as fuel, will attain the spiritual world, even if he is the most sinful of sinful persons, and the person who lights up that fire, will be freed from all sinful reactions…

Every part of the plant is fragrant—the leaves, seeds, and flowers. When in bloom, the fragrance of the tulsi is keenly felt. The plant seeds profusely. Natural regeneration is profuse.

On the banks of the Yamuna River is the religious city of Mathura, a city is associated with Krishna—the Hindu god who is regarded as an incarnation of Vishnu. Along the banks of this river during my work as a forest officer, I came across a patch of Ocimum sanctum bushes growing in the wild. We were exploring the prospects of establishing a nature park in which local species would be given a place of prominence. The intent was to create a nature park opposite the famous Mughal monument Taj Mahal which is located on the banks of the Yamuna River in the neighboring jurisdiction of Agra. At the time of this visit, the plants were in bloom and the air wasfull of fragrance— no wonder Hindus find the plant enchanting. As far as I can recall, the area had been enclosed and put under protection by the local forest officials to prevent the site getting damaged.

There are three varieties of the plant. Two of these are named after the Hindu gods Krishna and Rama—Krishna Tulsi and Rama Tulsi. The former has purple-tinged leaves and the latter is mostly green. A third variety—Van Tulsi ("van" in Sanskrit means "forest")—grows in the wild. All three varieties have similar aromatic and medicinal properties.

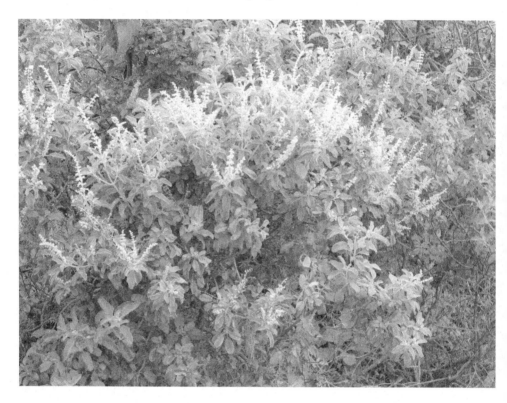

Picture 4: Ocimum tenuiflorum
Photo: Dr Ravikumar, Senior Botanist, FRLHT

The botanical name of the plant today is Ocimum tenuiflorum; the earlier name was Ocimum sanctum. Holy Basil should not be confused with Ocimum basilicum or common basil which is used as a spice in Mediterranean and European cuisine.

Holy Basil is indigenous to South Asia, cultivated widely in tropical regions of South and Southeast Asia. The plant has a clove-like peppery flavor and grows as an herb or a small shrub. It rarely grows to a height beyond two meters.

As Medicine

Tulsi is traditionally viewed as a plant that brings tranquility to the mind, assisting in meditation and concentration. It is regarded as a life-saving herb and is often referred to as "the elixir of life."

The herb is mentioned in Charakasamhita. There are monographs of O. tenuiflorum published in the Ayurvedic Pharmacopoeia of India (Vol. II, 1999, and Vol. IV, 2004), Unani Pharmacopoeia of India (Vol. V, 2008), Thai Herbal Pharmacopoeia (Vol. I, 1995), Vietnamese Pharmacopoeia (1st ed., 1983), and World Health Organization (WHO) Monographs (Vol. 2, 2002). Most of these systems of medicine recommend the use of the Holy Basil to treat arthritis, respiratory ailments, fever, influenza, stomach ailments, etc. Tulsi is a common ingredient in many Ayurveda and Unani medicines.

In India, it is a common home remedy for cold, cough, fever, influenza, etc. The leaves are brewed as a tea with a bit of garlic and cinnamon added to the decoction. Masala tea, popular in South Asia, is made by brewing tea with tulsi, garlic, black pepper, and cinnamon resulting in a uniquely strong spicy flavor.

Holy basil is an ingredient in Ayurvedic cardio-tonics, and cough, cold, and digestion aid medication. Ocimumosides A, B, and ocimarin are three compounds isolated from extract of leaves of holy basil that were proven to have anti-stress effects.

The anti-stress properties of the herb have been validated in multiple studies (Archana et al., 2002; Samson et al., 2006; Samson et al. (2007 and Ravindran et al., 2005). Its neuroprotective properties have been observed in multiple studies too (Yanpallewar et al., 2004; and Siddique et al., 2007).

The antioxidant properties of tulsi was observed by Subramanian et al., 2013) and), who also observed that it caused a reduction in oxidative stress in the brain. It was noted that tulsi possesses an amelioration property when the sciatic nerve was cut to induce neuro dysfunction in rats (Muthuraman et al., 2008). This property could have value in finding treatments in the dysfunctions caused by damage to the nerves.

Tulsi helps in normalizing hyperglycemia, plasma corticosterone, plasma creatine kinase, and adrenal hypertrophy (Gupta et al., 2007; Sembulingam et al., 2005; Sen et al., 1992; and Archana et al., 2000). Experiments on rabbits show that holy basil reduced lipid levels (Geetha et al., 2004). Lipid reduction and antioxidant property was also observed in another study (Manikandan et al., 2007). Cardioprotective property of the herb was observed and results published in another study (Mohanty et al., 2006).

A number of studies have been conducted to examine the role of Ocimum sanctum in treating diabetes (Kapoor, 2008). This study showed that it is effective in preventing insulin resistance. A similar property was observed in experiments on rats (Reddy et al., 2008). The leaves of the herb partially attenuated glycogen content and modulated carbohydrate metabolism in rats (Vats et al., 2004). Anti-diabetic properties were also observed in multiple studies (Hannan et al., 2006; and Agrawal et al., 1996).

The action of the herb against multiresistant strains of gonorrhea-causing organisms has been studied and validated (Shokeen et al., 2008; and Shokeen et al., 2005). The action of holy basil as a chemo preventive medicine has also been studied and validated (Nayak et al., 2005; Dutta et al., 2007; and Manikandan et al., 2007). The herb was also found to have a protective impact against induced skin tumors on experimental mice (Rastogi et al., 2007). The plant was observed to possess radioprotective, anti-carcinogenic, and antioxidant properties (Uma Devi, 2001). The oil from the seed was found to possess chemo preventive properties (Prakash et al., 2000).

Anti-ulcer and ulcer-healing properties of the herb were also observed

(Dharmani et al., 2004; Goel et al., 2005; Kath et al., 2006; and Singh et al., 1999). Vasudevan et al. (2001) studied its action against enteric pathogens. The plant was found to possess a reversible anti-fertility effect on experiments conducted on rats (Ahmed et al., 2002).

The plant contains alkaloids, glycosides, phenols, saponins, tannins, terpenes, etc. Various studies aimed at providing a modern scientific basis for its use in Ayurvedic medicine have been conducted by various Ayurveda medicine manufacturers in India. Dabur Pharmaceuticals, an India-based manufacturer of Ayurvedic medicine, claims that they conducted a trial on humans to validate the immune-modulatory effects of basil.

Several Ayurvedic drug manufacturers in India and abroad include the holy basil as a critical ingredient in preparations of organic teas.

The extensive use of the plant in India and its wide-scale cultivation and use in the production of a multitude of products indicate that the medicinal properties of the plant have caught the popular imagination of people. However, human trials need to be conducted to formalize the use of the herb as medicine.

I, too, have self-administered holy basil leaves to ease cold, cough, and flu symptoms and have found the herb's action soothing. This view, however, could be more a reflection of a mindset that has been passed on down through generation of Hindus or may be regarded as a placebo effect.

Scientific studies have just begun to probe some of the traditionally understood wonders of the plant. Perhaps, as the WHO (World Health Organization) has recommended, there is a need to study and analyze nature-based medicine systems separate from modern medical systems to truly leverage these wonders.

There are references to medicinal properties of holy basil in Chinese medicine too. Stomach spasms, kidney ailments, promotion of blood circulation, cuts, and inflammation are treated with holy basil. It is also believed to possess analgesic properties as per experiments conducted on mice (Khanna et al., 2003).

There are some references to the use of holy basil in Ancient Egypt, Greece, and Rome, but these may not be accurate as it is likely that it has been confused with the basil plant found in the region.

In Cosmetics

An essential oil is extracted from the leaves of the plant, mostly through the steam distillation process. The oil is rich in eugenol, nerol, camphor, and a variety of terpenes and flavonoids. These impart a clove-and-camphor-like aroma with a minty/lemony flavor. The presence of camphene, a bicyclic monoterpene, is the cause of the cooling feeling felt when a product containing holy basil is applied to the skin.

Tulsi oil diluted with carrier oils like olive or almond can be applied topically to the face or the body to ameliorate internal and external skin disorders. The oil has been proven to possess antibiotic, disinfectant, and antibacterial properties and is, for these reasons, used in small quantities in skin-conditioners, shampoos, and skin lotions.

A blend containing tulsi, lemon, and geranium oils is used in room fresheners and helps clear the lungs, like eucalyptus oil.

Estimates show annual Indian domestic consumption of holy basil to be over 3,500 metric tons. Most of this consumption is met by domestic sources. Holy basil is commercially cultivated by several international and Indian companies.

CHAPTER III

Indian sacred trees and their little-known health-giving properties

Ancient societies lived in harmony with nature, the source of food, medicine, and shelter. Religious and other texts contain references to ecology, trees, and animals as the worship of gods was associated with nature and trees. Traditions and folklore developed around nature, and certain trees were considered sacred.

It is only natural that India, a country that is sunny and hot for most of the year, considers large trees with dense foliage sacred. Peepal and banyan (Ficus religiosa and Ficus benghalensis) fall in this category. Mango (Mangifera indica) is not only a large tree with dense foliage but also yields luscious fruit, as is Bel-Aegle marmelos. Saraca indica, commonly known as Ashoka, has beautiful showy red flowers and is a sacred tree for the Hindus. In ancient Hindu texts, many other herbs and shrubs possessing medicinal or aromatic properties have also been declared sacred.

Vrukshayurveda, the science of plant life, is a 10th-century treatise ascribed to Surapala, and dealt with various species of trees and their growth. The verses of this treatise mention in some detail suitability of trees and plants in various ecosystems, their medicinal and other uses.[11]

The earliest reference to the worship of trees in India goes back to the Indus Valley Civilization (roughly the period of 2600-1800 BC). Seals from that era show people praying to a peepal tree.

Vedas, regarded as one of the holiest scriptures of the Hindus, were scripted by the Aryans.[12] A whole body of philosophical and religious

---

11   (http://www.indianscience.org/essays/t_es_agraw_surapala.shtml)
12   Some scholars claim that Aryans were people who migrated from regions close to the Arctic Circle in Russia bordering Central Asia. Others say that they were indigenous to India.

work was produced by these Vedic people. These include the Upanishads, the Upvedas like Ayurveda and epics like Ramayana and Mahabharata, and religious texts like Bhagwad Gita.

Many of these works allude to trees and plants. Manu, considered an early architect of the Hindu religion, has stated that trees are like humans and feel pleasure and pain. Eulogies to trees have been sung by various Indian sages and philosophers.

Wood of sacred trees like bel (Aegle marmelos), banyan (Ficus bengalensis), palasa (Butea monosperma), and peepal (Ficus religiosa) is not used as fuel even today by Hindus as it might invite the wrath of the gods. However, these trees did form an integral part of ancient sacrificial rites and ceremonies.

Trees have been associated with various gods in the Hindu religion. Aegle marmelos (bel), Zizyphus jujube (ber), and Elaeocarpus (rudraksa) are associated with Shiva; Ficus religiosa (peepal) and kadamba (Anthocephalus kadamba) are associated with Vishnu and his incarnate Krishna; mango with Hanuman the monkey god; ashoka to Kamadeva, the god of love; silk cotton (Bombax malabaricum) to Goddess Lakshmi[13]; and coconut to Varun the god of the waters. Hindu texts provide instructions on where each of these trees should be planted, when they should be worshipped, and which festivals are appropriate for their worship.

Trees have an important role in many Hindu rituals. A ceremonial pavilion is prepared with banana trunks as welcoming gates, and mango leaves are strung on door entrances at auspicious locations. The leaves of peepal and other Ficusspecies like Ficus glomerata (gular), Ficus lacor (pilkhan), Ficus benghalensis, and mango are used in prayers and offerings. Leaves of trees like wood apple (bel) are customarily offered to Lord Shiva; banana and arjuna (Terminalia arjuna) offerings are made to Ganesha (the elephant god).

---

13 Shiva, Vishnu, and Brahma form the Holy Trinity in Hindu religion. Their spouses are Parwati, Laxmi, and Saraswati.

Kautilya, a Brahmin guru, politician, and thinker (370-278 BC), laid down that those who cut even small branches or sprouts of trees yielding fruit and flowers, or providing shade in parks, places of pilgrimage, hermitage, and cremation or burial grounds, should be sternly dealt with. The Brhat Parasara Smrti states that he who plants and nurtures peepal, neem, margosa (Azadirachta indica), Ficus benghalensis, wood apple, myrobalan, mango, or tamarind trees will never see hell.

Human society all over the world has had a strong association with nature, as evidenced by the Biblical references to the Garden of Eden and those to plants and herbs in the Vedas. The cultural interaction between the Vedic and before them the Indus Valley Civilization and people of Greece, Mesopotamia, Sumeria, and Rome had an influence on the thinking of the time.[14]

Man has also been fascinated with the planets, the cycle of night and day, the sun, and the moon. He linked planetary movements to the destiny of nations, emperors, and individuals. The Vedanga Jyotisa, c. 1200 BC, is the earliest of the works about Vedic astronomy. Astronomy attributes were applied for timing social and religious events. There existed an intimate religious connection between astronomy and astrology at that time.

Ancient Hindu, Jain, and other literature associates astrology and plants. Herbal medicine and astrology were connected in the works of ancient Greek physicians and philosophers starting from Ptolemy, Hippocrates, and Galen down to Islamic scholar Avicenna. Each planet is associated with a plant, and each planet is considered to have an impact on the human body.

---

14   Greek astronomy ideas entered into India c. 4th century BC following the foray of Alexander in the Northwest region of India. This influence endured for over the millennia in India. Abul Fazl, the courtier of Akbar (15th century AD), wrote the seminal work on Akbar which contains reference to the preparation of the horoscope of baby Akbar using Greek astrological practices. Texts like Yavanajataka and Romaka were written in the early centuries of the Common Era. Aryabhata (c. 476-550 AD) was one of the earliest astronomer mathematicians whose works have survived over time. His work has had profound influence on the development of Islamic astronomy. Other famous mathematicians and astronomers of that age were Varahamihira (c. 550 AD), Bhaskara 1 (c. 629 AD), and Brahmagupta (c. 598-665 AD).

Planets affect all living beings, and herbs were used to calm, destroy, or reduce the malefic effects on humans. The most common example is the movement of the sunflower with the movement of the sun. The opening and shutting of many flowers is linked to the diurnal cycle. Hence, the ancient astrological view that plants are best collected during a period that corresponds to a planetary movement.

It was believed that the administration of medicine, if done during the time of day when the planetary effect is calculated to be most optimum on the Earth, will lead to early recovery. Both in Hindu and European astrology, different planets are associated with various plants.

Examples of association of planets with plants as per the Hindu belief are as follows:

Sun   Arka – Calatropis gigantean and wood apple tree or bael
   (Aegle marmelos)
Moon   Dhak – Butea monosperma and Manilkara hexandra (khirni)
Mars   Khaira – Althaea officinalis (marsh mallow) and Hemidesmus
   indicus (Indian sarasaparilla)
Mercury Apamarga – Achyranthes aspera or devils horsewhip
   and Argyreia speciosa (Vidhara)
Jupiter   Peepal – Ficus religiosa and banana root (Musa sps)
Venus   Gular – Ficus glomerata
Saturn   Shami – Prosopis cineraria
Rahu   Durva – Cynodon dactylon
Ketu   Kush – Cannabis indica and Sandalwood tree

Under the Ayurvedic system of medicine, remedies to alleviate malefic planetary effects have been described in detail.

A comparable association is also noted in the European herbal-cum-astrological system:
   The Sun: palm, rosemary, heliotrope, crocus, and all aromatics

The Moon: cucumber, gourd, pepin fruits, apples, pears, and lettuce
Mercury: corylus and millefoil
Venus: olive, pine, lily, rose, and pea
Mars: pepper, ginger, mustard, jalap, colocynth, euphorbium, all
bitter plants, and hot poisons
Jupiter: laurel, sandalwood, cinnamon, balsam, and the incense tree
Saturn: oak, rue, and generally all those of slow growth, of narcotic
virtue, and of crass substance

References to sacred trees are found in Shamanic, Hindu, Egyptian, Sumerian, Toltec, Mayan, Norse, Celtic, and Christian traditions. The tree of life is described in The Katha Upanishad as "a tree eternally existing, its roots aloft, and its branches spreading below." This is a description of a tree with prop roots. An example of such a tree is Ficus benghalensis. Many trees found in mangrove ecosystems would also fit this description.

In India, Ficus religiosa, banyan, and coconut are examples of trees that have been worshipped since time immemorial. Likewise, the Christmas tree is mentioned in Germanic mythology, the tree of knowledge (Kabbalah) in Judaism and Christianity, and the oak in the Celtic and the Druids. When we describe some of the trees revered in Hindu religion, we will notice that there exist philosophic similarities with those in other major religions of the world as well.

Sacred groves are woods of special religious and cultural importance to a community. Such woods are found across the world. In India too, most sacred groves are associated with an indigenous community belief in divinity of nature and natural resources. Some Indian sacred groves are truly ancient, going back to pre-Vedic times. Each of the groves is associated with a presiding deity or an ancient burial ground, which need not necessarily have an association with a mainstream religion.

The protection provided to sacred groves by the local communities has helped prevent endemic vegetation from disappearing. The degree of protection offered varies from grove to grove—in some groves, the communities-incharge do not permit even the dry foliage and fallen fruits to be touched. People believe that any kind of disturbance will offend the local deity, triggering disease, natural calamities, or failure of crops. In others, planting of new fruit trees like mango or neem (Azadirachta indica) is undertaken. There are around 14,000 sacred groves spread across India, spread across several kinds of ecosystems in the country.

According to Hindu tradition, forests were divided into three types: Tapovan, Mahavan, and Sreevan. Tapovan forests were meant for saints for meditation, and Mahavan were the grand, rich forests. Both forbade entry to local communities. Sreevan were used to meet the need for fuel, fodder, and timber.

This classification has some parallels to the classification of forests used in India today where the "reserve forests" are barred to human communities. In the "protected forests," some rights to local communities do exist, but most local needs are met from the village or community forests.

Sacred groves have acted as a natural repository for various Ayurvedic medicines. They are replenishable sources of honey and fruit, provide soil cover, help protect water bodies, and improve the local eco-climate. With increase in population and other biotic pressures, human need for infrastructure development, and the increased diminution of the importance of old deities, religious, and cultural practices, these islands of conserved habitat are under existential threat.

While there are many sacred groves across the length and breadth of India, perhaps the most well-known from the socio-religious standpoint could be the Lumbini Grove in Nepal. Lumbini is just across the International India-Nepal border in Nepali territory. The region is famous for its pristine Shorea robusta(sal) and deciduous forests. This grove was declared a World Heritage site by UNESCO in 1997 and marks the birth place of Gautama Buddha (c. 623-543 BC), the founder of Buddhism.

Sudhir Ahluwalia

Ficus religiosa- the tree that Hindus worship

For Hindus, this is perhaps the most sacred of all trees. In the Bhagavad Gita, Krishna says:

> Of all trees I am the Peepal tree, and of the sages among the demigods I am Narada. Of the Gandharvas I am Citraratha, and among perfected beings I am the sage Kapila.

Called ashvattha in Sanskrit, the peepal (Ficus religiosa) is a mid-to-large-sized tree. The species grows across the whole of South Asia and Southeast Asia. Its bark is light grey, smooth, and peels in patches. Its heart-shaped leaves have long, tapering tips that rustle in the slightest breeze. The fruit, when ripe, is purple in color.

History and Religious Overview

A seal from the Indus Valley Civilization period, discovered from Mohenjodaro, depicts a woman praying before what appears to be a peepal tree. The Brahma Purana and the Padma Purana, relate how, once when the demons defeated the gods, Vishnu found refuge in the thick foliage of a peepal tree. Praying to a peepal tree is thus equated with worshipping Vishnu. Worshipping trees reflect the ancient man's integral connection with nature.

In Hindu folklore, the peepal is a tree in which resides the Hindu Trinity of Shiva, Vishnu, and Brahma. Brahma is said to reside in the roots, Shiva in the leaves, and Vishnu in the trunk. The Skanda Purana also considers the peepal a symbol of Vishnu as in his human incarnation,[15] he is believed to have born and died under this tree.

---

15   In Hindu mythology, God takes birth as a human whenever evil forces start dominating the planet. In his human form, he destroys evil, restoring the balance. The incarnations of Vishnu include Rama, Krishna, and others.

In the Upanishads, the difference between the body and the soul is compared to the fruit of the peepal. The body is like the fruit which, being outside, feels and enjoys things. The soul is compared to a seed, which is inside and witnesses everything. According to the Skanda Purana, even if one does not have a son, the peepal can be treated as as one. It goes on to say that as long as the tree lives, the family name will continue.

Cutting a peepal tree is considered a sin comparable to killing a Brahmin, one of the five deadly sins, or Panchapataka. According to the Skanda Purana, any person who cuts a peepal tree would go straight to hell. The peepal tree symbolizes enlightenment and peace. People tie threads of white, red, and yellow silk around it in prayer for healthy progeny and rewarding parenthood.

The peepal is sacred to Buddhists too. The progeny of the ancient Bodhi tree (c. 288 BC) under which Buddha attained enlightenment still survives at Bodh Gaya, one of the most important pilgrimage centers of Buddhism. According to the Buddha, "He who worships the Peepal tree will receive the same reward as if he has worshipped me in person."

In a thickly populated country like India where land is at a premium, the religious significance accorded to trees is sometimes exploited to encroach public lands. The technique adopted is simple—tie a sacred red thread around the tree, place a few idols of Hindu gods under it, and call the place a temple. Over time, a temporary and, subsequently, a permanent structure is constructed on the site. Law enforcement officials, for fear of public backlash, rarely evict such encroachers.

Leaves of the tree are relished by elephants, camels, goats, and cattle. The leaf contains 10-14% protein and is ideal as nutritious silage for animals. Even though the tree is worshipped and valued as a shade tree across India, protecting these in public areas is tough. Cattle grazers subject these trees to severe lopping to feed cattle, goats, and other animals.

Efforts made to plant the tree as an ornamental shade-giving tree along roads in India, consequently, have achieved only partial success. Biotic pressures are mainly responsible for this observed poor success. The extensive foliage makes the tree a great sanctuary for birds, bats, etc.

The tree is an important host to lac-producing insects. Sticks of the tree's wood, when struck against each other, generate friction. The sparks generated can be used to light a fire.

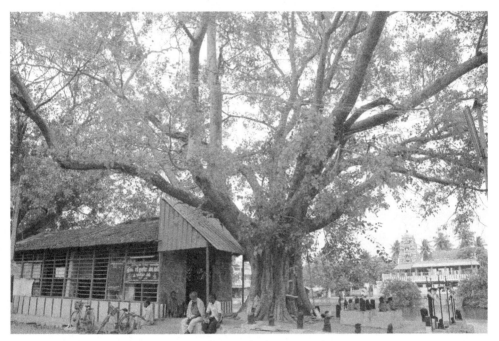

Picture 5 Ficus religiosa tree leaves
Photo: Dr Ravikumar, Senior Botanist, FRLHT

In Medicine

The peepal is valued in Ayurveda. It belongs to a class of drugs called rasayana—rejuvenators, antioxidants, and relievers of stress. The tree is also popular in Siddha, Unani, and homeopathic forms of medicine.

Various parts of the plant including the stem and root bark, aerial roots, vegetative buds, leaves, fruit, and latex are used to treat diseases like diabetes, vomiting, burns, gynecological ailments, dysentery, diarrhea, and nervous disorders (Prasad et al., 2006).

The tree is a tonic and astringent. Chemical analysis of the bark has identified presence of tannins, saponins, flavonoids, steroids, terpenoids, and cardiac glycosides. The molecules have medicinal properties. The bark has 4% tannin and is used to tan leather (Makhija et al., 2010).

The leaves have been proven to possess analgesic and anti-inflammatory properties (Gulecha et al., 2011). Experiments on guinea pigs revealed that extracts from the peepal fruit have a bronchospasm potentiating effect (Ahuja et al., 2011). The plant was, however, ineffective in controlling histamine-induced bronchial spasms. The traditional view that the tree could be effective in treating asthma was also demonstrated to be untrue in this experiment.

Leaves were observed to possess anti-amnesiac and memory-enhancing properties in experiments on rodents (Dewi et al., 2011; and Kaur et al., 2010). Hypolipidemic and antioxidant properties were observed in high fat induced hypercholesterolemia rats (Hamed, 2011). The bark was shown to possess anti-diabetic action in trials on rats (Pandit et al., 2010).

The traditional anti-ulcer medicinal properties of the bark were validated in an experiment conducted by Khan et al. (2011) on rats. Another study by Saha et al. (2010) validates the anti-ulcer potential of the plant.
Aerial root extracts were observed to possess anti-convulsant activity (Patil et al., 2011), as were the fruits (Singh et al., 2009).

The wound-healing potential of the leaf extracts of Ficus religiosa has been validated by an experiment conducted on rats (Roy et al., 2009). The anti-inflammatory and analgesic activity of the bark was also studied and validated (Sreeleksmi et al., 2007; Verma et al., 2010; and Viswanathan et al., 1990). Yadav et al. (2011) showed that the latex of Ficus religiosa has a preventive and curative effect against cispatin-induced nephrotoxicity in wistar rats.

Ayurvedic medicine with peepal as an ingredient is manufactured and sold in India. These claim to treat respiratory, digestive, and other ailments. The use of the plant in homeopathy has been studied, and clinical trials to study the efficacy of the plant in treating respiratory and digestive ailments have been conducted (Dey et al., 2008). The drug is used to treat hemorrhages of many kinds like hematemesis, menorrhagia, hemoptysis, etc.

Ficus benghalensis - tree with a thousand trunks

Banyan is one of the giant fig trees of India. These trees are known to live for hundreds of years. According to Bar-Ness, the banyan tree at Thimmamma Marrimanu, a village in Andhra Pradesh, ranks first in canopy cover (19,107 square meters). With a canopy area of 17,520 square meters is the second-largest banyan tree. The tree can be seen in a place called Kabir Vad in the Western Indian state of Gujarat

India's giant banyans find mention in the work of the Roman scholar Pliny (23-79 AD). In his Naturalis Historia, he describes the superlative canopy area of the "Indian fig tree" thus: "The upper branches spring, like a forest, from the vast body of the mother tree: most of them measure sixty paces in circumference; and they cover a space of two stadia with their shadow."

Pliny's knowledge of the giant Indian banyans came from Alexander's army, which sought refuge under a banyan tree on the outskirts of Bharuch in Gujarat. The army of 7,000 men is believed to have been sheltered under the broad and intricately linked branches of this great tree. This location is attributed to Kabir Vad where currently stands another giant banyan tree that is said to be over 300 years old.

The banyan tree in the National Botanical Garden at Kolkata covers an area of one and a half hectare with 2,880 prop roots and finds a place in the Guinness Book of Records as one of the largest trees in the world. The tree is estimated to be 250 years old. Both peepal and banyan are epiphytes. The plant can be seen sprouting in the crevices of buildings and attached to old walls.

The banyan tree finds figurative mention in the Bhagwad Gita:

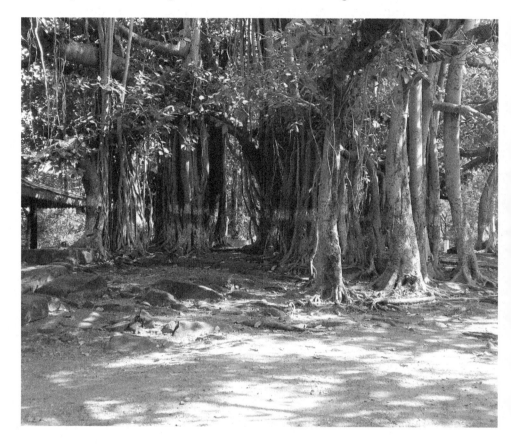

Picture 6 Banyan tree
Photo: Sudhir Ahluwalia

There is a banyan tree which has its roots upward and its branches down, and the Vedic hymns are its leaves. One who knows this tree is the knower of the Vedas.

(Bhagwad Gita 15.1)

The tree is mentioned in many scriptures as a tree of immortality. This is attributed to its aerial roots that have, over time, become additional trunks providing nourishment to the tree. The main trunk dies and decays over time, and the prop roots take over its functions.

As more prop roots develop and strike root into the ground, the surface area of the tree increases. In Hindu scriptures like the Gita, Upanishads, and the Puranas, in addition to epics like the Mahabharata, the tree is described as Bahu–pad (multiple feet). The shade of the banyan or peepal trees serves as a community meeting place in rural India.

Banyan has been traditionally planted along roads and around temples in India. The dense shade from the thick foliage provides relief in the hot summer months. These trees are a favorite resting place for humans, birds, and monkeys. The tree is easy to propagate vegetatively.

In Medicine

The species finds mention as medicine in Ayurveda, Siddha, Unani, and homeopathy. It is widely used in the treatment of diabetes. In the Unani system of medicine, the latex is regarded as an aphrodisiac and anti-inflammatory medicine. It is said to treat digestive ailments like dysentery and ulcers, biliousness, and serves as a tonic and astringent.

In Ayurveda, the banyan plant is used to treat skin diseases, vaginal disorders, leucorrhoea, menorrhea, and deficient lactation. A milky, sticky latex oozes from any injury on the plant. The latex is externally applied on bruises for relief. It relieves the pain. It is also used for relief in cases of rheumatism, back pain, and toothache. Leaves are heated and applied as a poultice to provide relief in abscesses. The bark is astringent, and the seeds have a cooling effect.

The Ayurvedic Pharmacopoeia of India recommends use of the aerial root in lipid disorders. The latex of the tree is also helpful in treating dysentery and diarrhea. The root bark, which contains ß-sitosterol, a D-glucose and meso-inositol, has anti-diabetic properties which can treat pituitary and alloxan-induced diabetes. Hypoglycemic action of a glucoside (bengalenoside) isolated from Ficus benghalensis was demonstrated to be effective against normal and alloxan diabetic rabbits (Augusti, 1975).

Extract from the roots of the tree were found to stimulate cell and antibody mediated immune responses in rats. It enhanced the phagocytic function of human neutrophils in-vitro (Gabhe et al., 2006). Antimutagenic and antioxidant activity of stem bark of Ficus benghalensis and root extract of Moringa oleifera was seen in a study conducted by Satish et al. (2013).

The hypolipidemic and antioxidant property of the bark of the banyan tree was observed in rabbits (Shukla et al., 2004). The bark of the tree was found to possess anti-stress and anti-allergic properties (Taur et al., 2007). Anti-helminthic activity of the species was seen by Aswar et al. (2008). The anti-microbial activity of the roots and the fruit extract was seen in studies conducted by Murti et al. (2011) and Gaherwal (2013).

Ethanolic and aqueous extracts of F. benghalensis have properties that promote accelerated wound-healing activity. This property was observed in placebo control trials. The wound- healing property of F. benghalensis may be attributed to the presence of phyto-constituents in the plant (Garg et al., 2011). The anti-inflammatory activity of the plant on rats was observed in experiments conducted by Deore et al. (2012).

Significant anti-helminth action of banyan tree aerial roots has been studied and validated (Tuse et al., 2011). The anti-microbial action of the plant has also been studied and validated against a range of disease-causing bacteria like Escherichia coli, Klebsiella sps, etc. (Ogunlowo et al., 2013). The antioxidant and anti-mutagenic properties of the plant have also been studied by scientists.

Aegle marmelos – fruits that tone the digestive system

The mid-sized wood apple tree (botanical name Aegle marmelos) is of immense religious significance to Hindus. Leaves and fruit are offered in worship to Shiva, one of the gods of the Hindu Trinity. Hindus believe that Shiva resides in the Bael (Aegle marmelos) tree. The trifoliate leaves of the species are said to represent the three eyes of Shiva.

The tree is mentioned in Yajur Veda. Varahamihira (505-587 AD), the ancient mathematician and author, mentions Aegle marmelos in his encyclopedic work, Brihat Samhita. Brihat Samhita covers a range subjects including astrology, astronomy, rainfall, clouds, architecture, growth of crops, manufacture of perfume, matrimony, domestic relations, gems, pearls, and rituals.

The species finds a mention in ancient Buddhist texts too. The tree is part of a fertility ritual in Nepal. Young girls, in devotion to God Shiva, tie a thread around the Bael tree, consummating a cosmic marriage with the Lord. Hindu iconography has multiple references that associate the tree with God Shiva. The planting of this tree around a home or temple is said to sanctify the place. Ancient Sanskrit texts refer to its fruit as the fruit of prosperity. The Chinese Buddhist pilgrim, Xuanzang, who travelled extensively in India (6th century AD), mentions the Bael in his chronicles.

The species is found in South and Southeast Asia. In India, it thrives in the dry deciduous regions. It can survive a wide temperature range from -8 to 48 degrees Celsius.

The tree is usually grown near temples and rarely felled for timber or firewood. It is valued more for its fruit and other properties. The wood is yellowish or grayish white. It is a hardwood. It takes fine polish and can be used both in furniture and as small timber. The tree rarely acquires girth beyond one meter in diameter.

In India, the twigs are used used in this manner include as a natural tooth brush. Other herbs Acacia nilotica (common name: babul) and Azadirachta indica(common name: neem) trees. Chewing on these cleans the teeth and freshens the mouth.

The juice from the leaves helps remove foul odor from the body when applied before taking a wash. The unripe rind of the fruit yields a yellow dye. Along with myrobalans, the dye is used in calico printing. The fruit pulp has detergent properties and can be used as a substitute for soap. The stem yields a non-edible gum that can be used as an adhesive.

In Thailand and Indonesia, tender young leaves and shoots are used as a vegetable. An infusion of the flowers makes a cooling drink. The fruit casing is woody and hard and must be hammered open. Inside the ripe fruit lies a sweet pulp rich in fiber, calcium, potassium, phosphorus, iron, minerals, and vitamins A, B1, C, and riboflavin.

The ripe fruits of wood apple are sold in the markets across India. During the summer months from May to July when dry, hot winds blow across the plains of North and Central India, a refreshing drink made from the sweet pulp of the fruit mixed with sugar and water provides relief to the body. Heat strokes and dehydration are common during this period, and the fruit makes for a popular cooling drink.

The fruit is a home remedy in cases of dyspepsia, indigestion, acidity, nausea and other forms of abdominal discomfort. The divinity attributed to this tree could be partly because of its multiple medicinal, nutritional, and other properties.

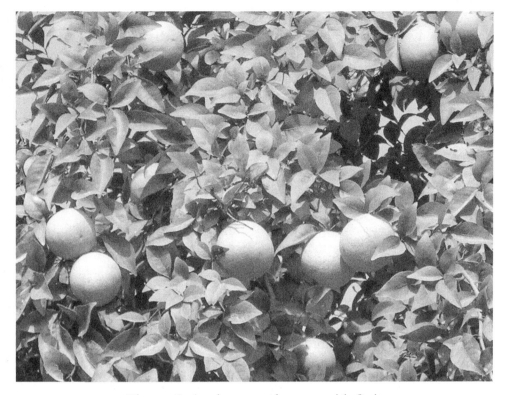

Picture 7: Aegle marmelos tree with fruit
Photo: Dr Ravikumar, Senior Botanist, FRLHT

In Medicine

Ayurvedic and other herbal healers recommend the fruit for relief in cases of jaundice, dysentery, diarrhea, constipation, and even ulcers. The plant's medicinal properties are accepted in nearly all the ancient medical systems including Ayurveda, Siddha, Unani, Chinese, tribal, Greek, and Roman (Ariharan et al., 2013). Ancient literature has documented medicinal properties of the leaves, bark, and roots. These benefit patients with gastroenterological ailments.

Aegle marmelos has been included on the WHO list of herbal drugs as well as the Ayurvedic Pharmacopoeia of India. In homeopathy, it is used for treating conjunctivitis, styes, rhinitis, coccygodynia, nocturnal seminal emission with amorous dreams, and chronic dysentery. Its leaves are used for fertility control in Bangladesh.

The unripe fruit is known to be effective against giardia and rotavirus of the gut and stomach (Baliga, 2011). Research studies have shown the effectiveness of the plant against 21 disease-causing bacteria and fungi that include Staphylococcus sps, Salmonella sps, Bacillus sps, Aspergillus sps, Klebsiella sps, etc. (Pandey et al., 2011).

Fruit extracts are seen to possess anti-genotoxic properties (Kaur et al., 2009). Studies conducted on rats indicate the hypoglycemic (anti-diabetic) property of Aegle marmelos (Upadhyay et al., 2004).

Jayachandraetal.(2009)observedinastudyonratsthatthehepatoprotective property of Aegle marmelos leaf extracts is comparable to the standard Liv52 drug. The action of the plant in containing hyperlipidemic conditions and its antioxidant properties were observed in an experiment conducted on rabbits fed a high-fat diet by Das et al. (2012). A study done by Singh et al. (2012) has also shown the anti-helminthic property of leaf extracts.

The anti-inflammatory effect of aqueous and methanol extracts of Aegle marmelos seeds was evaluated by Sharma et al. (2011) using carrageenan-induced paw edema and cotton pellets-induced granuloma in rats. They found that the aqueous extract also possessed significant ($P<0.05$) anti-inflammatory properties.

The Centre for Cellular and Molecular Platforms has developed the technology to produce Aegle marmelos (Bael) fruit extracts. These have been shown to possess a cytotoxic effect against tuberculosis causing bacteria, Mycobacterium tuberculosis. The antioxidant property of the fruit pulp was studied by Rajan et al. (2011).

The anti-ulcer property of the extracts was attributed to the presence of quercetin-like (Flavonoid) contents by Sharma et al. (2011). Rajeshkannan et al. concluded that the species possesses anxiolytic and anti-depressant properties.

Modern research has identified properties that could aid in the cure of cancer (George et al., 2014), HIV, and AIDS (Sabde et al., 2011). Phyto-constituents isolated from the plant include skimmianine, an alkaloid that has been indicated to possess an anti-cancer property. The plant protects normal tissue from chemicals and radiotherapy and could benefit patients who have undergone such treatments.

Healers prescribe plant extracts in combination with other plants like Azadirachta indica and Occimum tenuiflorum, two other sacred plants of India.

Anthocephalus kadamba – with flowers for lovers

Stanza 1 of Jayadeva's Gitagovindam, or "Song of Govinda," (a poetic work on Lord Krishna composed in 1200 AD) goes,

> "He who is mixed up or mingled in the darkness at a peaceful Kadamba tree, pre-set by me—deserve supreme love and affection of the Supreme and hence I reminisce about him."[16]

I have been fortunate to spend some time under a grove of Kadamba trees in full bloom while working at Mathura which is considered the birthplace of Krishna the Hindu God incarnate. It was a hot summer day when I, along with my team, visited a village for routine administrative work. The day, I remember, was sunny and hot, and the plains were as dry as a cake. In the distance, a grove of trees appeared, and the wind brought a waft of scent.

---

16   (http://eol.org/pages/1106567/details)

I enquired about the scent to the local officer accompanying me and was told that the grove in front of us— and we must be half a kilometer away from it—was a pure collection of Anthocephalus kadamba.

We stopped our vehicle under the shade of these trees; the air was full of fragrance, and the trees filled with yellow to orange globose flowers. It was indeed divine. The villagers had put a couple of cots under the shade of these trees; being a poor village, the people did not possess chairs or anything else. But the place was divine, and I cherish it, even after 25 years since I visited the place.

After this visit, we launched a drive to plant kadamba trees on all avenues around the famous Taj Mahal in Agra and across that city, but with limited success. Protecting trees from vandals in a city is a huge challenge. Unfortunately, the kadamba trees appear to be in danger of disappearing from the region.

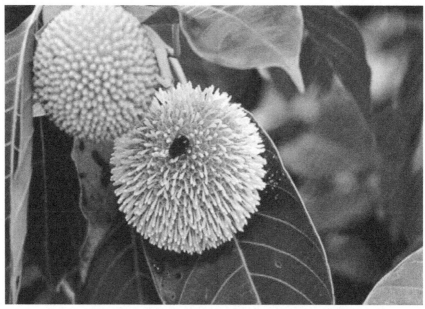

Picture 8 Anthocephalus cadamba flowers
Photo by Balaram Mahalder

In Hindu mythology, the tree was the favorite tree of Lord Krishna, who is depicted playing a flute under it. The tree is known as Haripriya or "God's favorite." It is a culturally and religiously significant tree in Java and Malaysia too. In the southern parts of India, the kadamba is regarded as the abode for the Goddess Durga, consort of Shiva, who is said to reside in a forest of kadamba.

There is a reference to the tree in the Bhagavata Purana. Kalidasa, the famous playwright (400-500 AD), mentions women wearing flowers of kadamba. Nowadays, Indian women prefer to wear other scented flowers, usually cultivated ones, like jasmine. The natural forests of kadamba are now restricted to a few groves or a few dispersed trees across the country and the availability of flowers is rare to infrequent.

The species is found not just in the dry northern plains of India, but also in the wet, semi-evergreen forests of the Western Ghats region in South India. Before the introduction of the ban on green felling by the Government of India, I remember that we would mark Anthocephalus kadamba trees in these forests for extraction by the plywood industry. The tree has a clean bole of nine meters or more and a tree height that could go up to 20-25 meters. Girths of two meters at breast height are common. Clean bole makes it ideal for peeling for plywood. The wood is also good to be converted into splints to make matches.

Kadamba veneers sold in the local market in India are largely of artificial synthetic origin in which the surface is designed to give it a natural look. Softwood like that from kadamba trees can be impregnated with synthetic resin to increase density and enhance strength. Such wood is used in furniture-making as well in the construction industry. In addition, a yellow dye is obtained from the root bark. With the discovery of chemical dyes, dyes from herbs, shrubs, and trees are no longer popular.

As Perfume

Kadamba flowers are used to make the Indian perfume that is locally called attar or ittr. The essential oil, extracted by steam distilling the flowers, is yellow in color and has a woody floral odor with a short-lived but strong minty borneol
top note.The tenacity of the perfume is incredible, according to Arctander, and the dry note is delightfully sweet-floral, reminiscent of Champaca and Neroli, two of the other popular Indian floral perfumes.

With the growing shortage of trees of kadamba, the oil has become more difficult to procure and the price has shot up. Kadamba is often blended with other natural perfumes, mainly sandalwood. Aromatherapists use kadamba attar to calm and relax the body.

In Medicine

The bark of the stem is used as medicine in Ayurveda, Siddha, and Unani systems. The Ayurvedic Pharmacopoeia of India mentions use of dried stem bark to treat female genital tract and bleeding disorders. Charaka (c. 200 BC) categorized it as an analgesic. The fruit pulp is described as a purifier of seminal fluids. Sushruta (his era is unclear and is put between 1200 BC and 600 BC) has cited it as a detoxifier and anti-diarrheal.

The traditional healers of the Bastar region in Central India use the bark of the kadamba to treat afflictions to the eye. It is also used to give relief in cases of inflamed and sore mouth (stomatitis). The traditional healers of Chhattisgarh Plains use a decoction made from the leaves as medicine.

The fruit juice treats gastric irritability in children. Anthocephalus cadamba is ethno-medically widely used in the form of a paste by tribes in the Western Ghats to treat skin diseases. The tribes of Ganjam district of the East Indian state of Orissa drink the root paste suspended in water to reduce blood sugar in cases of diabetes mellitus.

It is used as a folk medicine to treat fever, anemia, uterine complaints, blood diseases, skin diseases, leprosy, dysentery, and for improving the semen quality. The leaves are recommended as a gargle in cases of stomatitis. Indole alkaloids, terpenoids, sapo genins, saponins, terpenes, steroids, fats, and reducing sugars have been identified in the plant.

Anthocephalus cadamba stem bark is reported to possess tonic, astringent, febrifugal, and anti-diuretic properties. It is also used to treat cough. Juice from the bark, along with other compounds, is used to treat inflammation of the eye.

The anti-pyretic action of the plant was studied in trials on rats and the results found it comparable to the action of paracetamol (Usman et al., 2012). Anthocephalus cadamba bark extract has an anti-inflammatory agent, and a study conducted on rats proved this (Chandrashekar et al., 2010).

The dried bark is reported to contain steroids, alkaloids, fats, and reducing sugar. It is used to improve semen quality (Gurjar et al., 2010). A. cadambaleaves, extracted in chloroform, were studied for their cytotoxic effect on different human cancer cell lines (Singh et al., 2012). Nagakannan et al. (2011), in their animal trials with extracts, have observed that they have sedative and anti-epileptic properties. The alcoholic and aqueous extracts of fruits (ripened and un-ripened) of this plant showed significant antibacterial activity against many pathogens like Staphylococcus aureus, Escherichia coli, and Pseudomonas aeruginosa (Mishra et al. 2011).

The results of an experimental study conducted by Dubey et al. (2011) showed that it is possible to develop an anti-microbial ointment with alcoholic extract of Anthocephalus cadamba leaves. This can be useful in treating skin diseases caused by Escherichia coli (E. coli), Pseudomonas aeruginosa (P. aeruginosa), Staphyllococcus aureus (S. aureus), and Aspergilus niger (A. niger).

The hypoglycemic activity of the root was compared with the reference standard drug glibenclamide. The study revealed that the extract of the roots caused significant reduction in the blood glucose level in both normoglycemic and alloxan-induced diabetic rats (Acharaya et al., 2010). Its anti-diabetic properties have been studied by Alam et al. (2011).

Saraca asoca – evergreen tree for a healthy uterus

This is a mid- to small-sized evergreen tree found in the wet evergreen forests of the Western Ghats in South India. It is also observed in similar habitats in South and Southeast Asia. The trees bear showy red flowers. The enchanting beauty of the Ashoka in bloom has been described in many ancient Sanskrit verses including in the poetry written by the 5th century poet and playwright Kalidasa.

I, too, have witnessed the trees in bloom. As part of my professional duties, it was common for me, along with the local officers, to visit 50-
to even 100-year-old plantations of various species. These inspections were aimed to assess the condition of these forests and make decisions on management interventions required to improve their condition. As part of this routine exercise in one of the forest ranges—the Gersoppe Forest Range in the North Kanara district of Karnataka—the local range forest officer walked me into this stand that was a sea of red in the ocean of green of the evergreen forest.

This was a moister site when compared to the rest of the area, a pure stand. The forest floor under the Ashoka stand was richer and healthier when compared to the adjacent forest site made up of planted teak. Teak plantations in evergreen ecosystems often leads to deterioration of the site, making them drier.

Historical and Religious Overview

Ashoka is another of the sacred plants of Hindus, representing the Hindu god of Love, Kamadeva. The god and the tree are worshipped
every year on December 27. It is no wonder that there is a lot of folklore surrounding this tree.

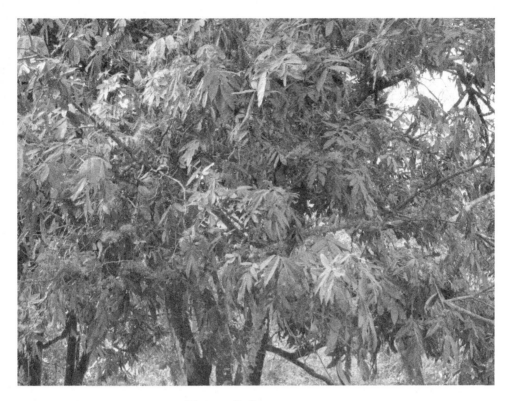

Picture 9: Saraca asoca
Photo: Dr Ravikumar, Senior Botanist, FRLHT

Hindus believe that the touch of the ashoka tree relieves a person of worries—one of the Sanskrit names for the species is nasty-soka or "reliever of worries." Padma Purana states, "The planting of asoka tree leads to the destruction of all sorrows." Varaha Mitra, in his encyclopedic work Vrhat Samhita, says that planting of asoka, siris (Albizzia lebbek), etc. in the garden or in the house brings welfare to the household.

Mythical stories on ashoka abound. One explains how the ashoka tree starts blooming at the touch of the female feet to which is attributed the name padaghatadasoka. Kalidasa, the poet who lived in the 4th century AD, describes the dance of Malvika, the courtesan under an ashoka tree, in his work Maavikagnimitram.

In Buddhism, too, the ashoka tree is associated with the incarnations of the Buddha. Xuan Zhang, a Chinese visitor to India in the 7th century AD, claims that the Buddha himself was born under an ashoka tree, though this is disputed by others who say that the birth happened under a sala tree (Shorea robusta). Indeed, if the Buddha's place of birth was Lumbini in Nepal, then the latter opinion is more possible as it is a region that abounds in sala trees and not ashoka.

The 2nd century BC stone railing discovered at Bharhut has a carving that depicts an ashoka tree intertwined with the figure of a goddess. Figures with similar association of goddesses with the ashoka tree are interpreted as the association of the tree with spirits of fertility spirits (Biswas and Debnath, 1972).

In Medicine

Charakasamhita has described ashoka's effects as an astringent and analgesic. It was used to treat skin diseases including leprosy. Sushruta, too, has stated that ashoka is an astringent. It was recommended as treatment for disorders of the womb. Other medicinal uses of ashoka are its use to treat wounds, snake bites, eye ailments, neurological disorders, and fever.

Ashokarishta is a popular Ayurvedic medicine. It is prescribed to treat premenstrual ailments. The bark of the ashoka tree is said to have a stimulating effect on the endometrium and the ovarian tissue. It is useful
 in all cases of uterine bleeding. It is also useful in menorrhagia due to uterine fibroids, in leucorrhea and in internal bleeding. Bark is stripped from the tree only after it has attained 10 years of age. The stripped bark is then sundried.

Methanolic extract of Saraca indica leaves (400 mg/kg) produced enhanced activity as a central nervous system depressant. This property was studied in cases of prolonged sleep duration induced by pentobarbitone. It decreased locomotor activity by 67.33% (Verma et al., 2010).

The anti-helmintic activity against adult earthworms (Pheretima posthuma) of leaf extracts from Saraca indica has been studied. At 40 mg/ml concentration, methanol extracts showed better anti-helminthic activity than the standard drug albendazole (Sharma et al., 2011). Anti-bacterial properties of leaf extracts were studied in 2011 by Nayak et al.

The cardio-protective effect of Saraca indica is attributed to its antioxidant activity (Swamy et al., 2013). The antioxidant properties of the stem bark were identified by Panchawat et al. (2010), along with the anti-diarrheal properties.

Experimental results show that the leaf extracts have significant anti-tumor and cytotoxic effect against the human cervical cancer HeLa cell line. This study supports the ethno-medical use of Saraca indica (Asokan et al., 2014). A study conducted by Verma et al. (2011) indicates that the leaf extracts of the plant has analgesic impact. Saraca asoca contains glycoside, flavonoids, tannins, and saponins.

Elaeocarpus ganitrus with psychotherapeutic fruits

The fruit of Elaeocarpus ganitrus is used to make a string necklace from the dried fruit beads. Rudraksha is the Sanskrit name of the seed which is used as Hindu prayer beads. The word "rudraksha" is made up of two words: "rudra" is the name given to Shiva, the Hindu god who is regarded as an incarnation of the destructive power of God, and "aksha" which translates to "eye" in Sanskrit.

It is a broad-leaved evergreen tree species found in the India's East Himalayan foothills (up to an altitude of 2,000 feet), Nepal, and in Southeast Asia. It grows as a giant tree reaching heights of up to 65 meters.

The tree starts producing fruits from its seventh year onward. Fruits fall to the ground when ripe and are collected from the forest floor. Each tree is known to yield one to two thousand fruits annually. To collect the fruit from the forest floor, the area under the tree is swept clean, an ecologically destructive process as it leaves no seeds and other flora at the foot of these trees. Natural regeneration does not occur as there are no seeds to germinate, leading to a steady diminution of numbers of this species in its natural habitat.

Nepal, Indonesia, and India are the three sources of rudraksha. Nearly 75% of rudraksha comes from Indonesia. The surface of the fruit of the Indonesian variety is relatively smooth and is preferred for making necklaces.

The Indian variety has the roughest surface with the Nepalese lying in between these two. The Nepalese rudraksha seeds are hard, compact, and lustrous. These are the most expensive and rare of the three varieties

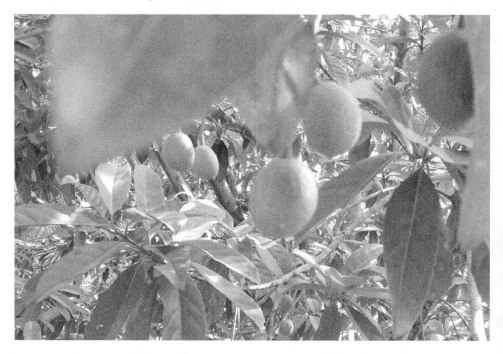

Picture 10 Elaeocarpus ganitrus tree
Photo: Sudhir Ahluwalia

The rudrakha beads are classified based on the number of furrows on the fruit surface; the more furrows, the more valued the bead is. The

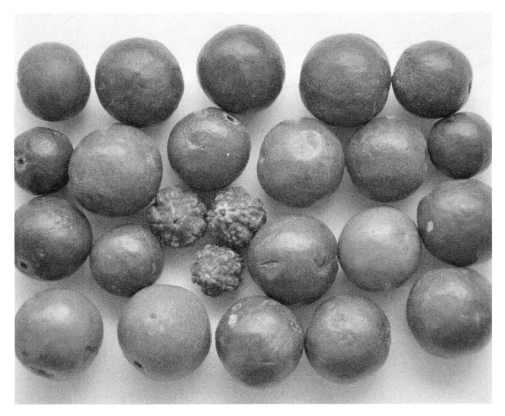

Picture 11 Rudraraksh (E. ganitrus) Fruit
Photo: Dr Ravikumar, Senior Botanist, FRLHT

Puranas[17] describe fourteen kinds of rudraksha. A rosary made from the beads is assigned a fixed set of auspicious numbers like 108+1, 54+1 and 27+1. An extra bead is placed as a marker or boundary from where the cycle begins again. This marker is not counted when chanting prayers.

---

17   Puranas are, for Hindus, one of the most important of the ancient Sanskrit texts. Wendy Doniger dates these texts from 250 CE to 1000 CE. These texts deal with a range of subject areas from mythology, cosmology, religion, astrology, geography, history, etc.

It is believed by many Hindus and Buddhists that the wearer of a necklace made of rudraksha beads is protected from negative influences. Indian astrologers use the rudraksha to remove malefic effects of the planets on an individual.

Astrological powers of the rudraksha is said to stem from the external indentation found on the fruit surface. There is a maximum of 14 indentations that can be found on a rudrarasksa fruit. The fruit that is astrologically most beneficial is the one that has a single face or indentation.

In Medicine

Shiva Purana, Padma Purana, and Bhagwat Gita refer to the greatness and healing powers of rudraksha. According to the Ayurvedic medical system, wearing rudraksha can have a positive effect on the heart and nerves. It helps relieve a person from stress, anxiety, depression, palpitations, and the lack of concentration. It is also used to treat nerve pain, epilepsy, migraine, asthma, hypertension, arthritis, and liver diseases. It is highly regarded for its anti-aging effect, and electromagnetic and inductive properties. People with high blood pressure claim benefit from the use of rudraksha seeds.

Rudraksha contains indolizidine type of alkaloids, minerals, vitamins, steroids, flavonoids, etc. Aqueous extract of leaves contains glycosides while an ethanolic extract contains gallic acid, ellagic acid, and quercetin.

A study conducted by Dr. Jayantha Kumar Sarma et al. (2010) on cats indicates that rudraksha has the potential to reduce hypertension. Another study on rats also indicates anti-hypertensive property of the species (Sakat et al., 2009). The anti-diabetic property has been observed in trials conducted on rats, and they showed that it is comparable to the modern drug glimepiride (Srikanth et al., 2012; and Juvekar et al., 2011)

Its anti-fungal property was found to be effective against Candida albicans and moderately effective against Aspergillus niger. The immuno-modulatory effect has also been identified in a study by Hule (2010). The antioxidant effect of the leaves was studied by Kumar et al.

(2008).

Leaf extracts exhibit a broad spectrum of anti-microbial activity. They were found to inhibit the growth of Staphylococcus aureus, Bacillus cereus, Escherichia coli, Pseudomonas aeruginosa, Klebsiella pneumoniae, Penicillium sp, Aspergillus flavus, Candida albicans, and C. tropicalis. The extract showed maximum relative percentage inhibition against B. cereus (Singh B et al., 2010).

Rudraksha Oil

Cold, compressed, 100% pure oil is extracted from rudraksha seeds. It is used as a dietary supplement. Ingesting two drops of oil a day is said to assist with internal healing. It is also used as hair oil as it helps remove dandruff, acts as a hair conditioner, and reduces acne and pimples. It helps pacify the skin conditions of eczema and ringworm, reducing the itching and speeding the healing of the skin. It is also used as a body massage oil.

Mango – the king of Indian fruits

The origin of the mango tree is believed by some to be in the Northeast hill region of India bordering Myanmar. Presence of mango tress in undisturbed forests in the interior of the Western Ghats region of South India, though, is evidence of a much wider native distribution.

Wild mango trees in semi-evergreen and evergreen habitats have clear boles, attain heights comparable to the tallest trees in the ecosystem, and have smaller leaves. The cultivated varieties are squat and well branched with relatively larger leaves.

Vedas and Puranas bear extensive references to the mango. The fruit was a valued source of food from the earliest of times and is hailed as the "king of fruits" and "food of the gods." The Hindu epics, Ramayana and Mahabharata, make multiple references to mango, reiterating the importance given to the fruit. The Greeks first encountered mango in India during the invasion by Alexander (c. 325 BC). There are references to Buddha meditating under a mango tree and relishing the fruit.

Selecting the best fruit-yielding wild mango trees was the initial means of genetic selection. This practice of plant selection probably continued for over 4,000-6,000 years. Cultivar improvement through vegetative propagation began probably about 400 years ago. Plant propagation was done vegetatively and not from seed.

History and Mythology

According to Hinduism, Prajapati, the progenitor and creator of all creatures, transformed himself into a mango tree. The Upanishads have dwelt on the concept of Prajapati in depth. I could not find a comparative analogy in other faiths and philosophies. Prajapati is not the earliest man (aka Adam or Eve). He could be better described as a creator of all things mortal.

Mango is also referred to as a King of Fruits. Establishing a mythical connection between this tree and Prajapati reflects the importance given to this tree by ancient man. Mythologically, this is how the story of the mango began. The earliest references to the mango go back to the Rigveda, the earliest of the Vedas, c. 1500 BC.

The Vedic people regularly lit sacred fires (yajnas) and chanted verses to propitiate the gods. Vessels containing sacred offerings used in Vedic yajnaswere adorned with mango leaves to represent the mythical pot containing elixir of immortality, amrit, or ambrosia.

There are references to the mango in Jain religion too. These go back to the 6thcentury AD. Mango is one of the five dev vrikhsha (tree of the gods). In Sanksrit poetry, mango is referred to as kalpa vriksha or "the wish granting tree."

Mango leaves, or its branches, are used in most Hindu rituals. A string of mango leaves is tied above the main entrance of a home celebrating an important event like a wedding, birth, religious festival, or any other event.

The mango is regarded as a symbol of love and life. In Kalidasa's (c. 4th century AD) writings, mango flowers are represented as the cupid's arrow. Mango in bloom symbolizes the onset of spring. Hieun Tsang, the Chinese scholar and traveler, also known as Xuanzhang, observed in the 6th century that mango played an important role in religious and social life of India.

Fruit and Production

The famous 14th century poet Amir Khusro refers to the mango in his poetry. The Mughal Emperor Akbar, who ruled large territories in the subcontinent in the 16th century, ordered that 100,000 mango trees be planted in Darbhanga, Bihar state, India. In the pre-industrial era, society was nearly wholly dependent on whatever the land could provide. Ordering planting of fruit orchards was a welfare measure aimed to provide food security to the people of a region.

Mango was introduced to the Middle East through trade. A vibrant trade, as we learned earlier, existed between India and this region at least since 2600 BC.
Mango is cultivated in tropical and subtropical regions across the globe, including Latin America, Florida in the US, Caribbean, Southeast Asian countries, South and Central Africa, Australia, and tropical parts of China.

India, China, and Thailand are the world's three largest producers of mango. Mango is the fifth most proliferate fruit in use in the world, with banana leading the pack. India accounts for 57.18% of total global production. Statistics have placed global production of mango in 2012 at 42.14 million metric tons.

Mango orchards in India are estimated to cover 1.6 million hectares of area. Annual fruit production ranges from 13-17 million metric tons. China comes next in production with around 4 million metric tons and Thailand follows with 2.5 million metric tons per annum.

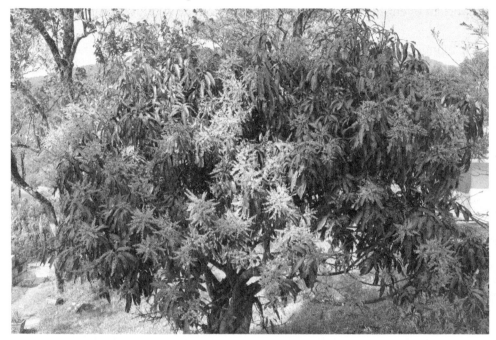

Picture 12 Mango tree in bloom
Photo: Dr Ravikumar, Senior Botanist, FRLHT

Nutrition and Food

There are over 400 varieties of mangoes and over 1,000 vegetatively propagated cultivars. Each cultivar has a unique flavor, sweetness, color, and taste. Mango is eaten both ripe and unripe, in pulp and juice form. It is also candied and converted into jam and nectar or is pickled. The unripe fruit of some varieties is particularly sour. Such fruit is sliced, dried, and ground to a powder used
to flavor curries.

Mango fruit is rich in sugar, low in fat, and contains vitamins, minerals, enzymes, and antioxidants. It is rich in potassium, calcium, iron, vitamin A and C, and fiber. They are an excellent source of beta-carotene and beta-cryptoxanthin. Both carotenoids are converted to active forms of vitamin. The total carotenoid count in mangoes rises with the ripening of the fruit. Since beta-cryptoxanthin is best absorbed by the body when eaten with fat, in order to maximize health benefits, mangoes are customarily consumed in India with milk and yoghurt.

Mango is an important food supplement in India. It fruits in summer when the production of vegetables gets depleted by the intense summer heat. Mango trees planted along roads and public spaces are a common source of high nutrition for birds, animals, and humans.

Ripe and unripe mangos are a good source of vitamin C. They contain an enzyme that aids in breaking down proteins, thus helping in the digestion process. The high iron content in the mango makes up for the deficiency created by menstruation and pregnancy. Potassium and magnesium micronutrients contained in the fruit alleviate muscle cramps, stress, acidosis, and prevents heart ailments.

The high insoluble fiber content in the fruit makes it a useful natural remedy in constipation. Tartaric and malic acids present in the fruit help in maintaining the alkali reserves in the body, balancing the pH value of the blood. The fruit is rich in antioxidants helping build immunity that can be further enhanced by flavonoids contained in the fruit.

The sap of the fruit contains a hazardous chemical named urushiol which can cause dermatitis. It is important, therefore, that the fruit is washed well before consuming.

In the hot summer months, a cooling drink—locally called panna—is prepared from unripe mango fruit to help prevent sunstrokes. Other home remedies include making a decoction from soaked young mango leaves to alleviate diabetes. A powder of mango kernel is used to strengthen gums. Dried flowers help treat dysentery and diarrhea. Juice of mango leaves helps relieve cough, and the ash helps relieve pain from wounds, etc.

In Medicine

Studies conducted on mango validate the traditional medicinal properties of the species like its anti-diabetic, antioxidant, anti-viral, cardiotonic, hypotensive, anti-inflammatory, antibacterial, anti-fungal, anti-helminthic, anti-parasitic, anti-tumor, anti-HIV, anti-bone resorption, anti-spasmodic, anti-pyretic, anti-diarrheal, anti-allergic, immune-modulation, hypolipidemic, anti-microbial, hepato-protective, and gastro-protective properties.

Experiments on rats conducted by Venkatalakshmi et al. (2011) have shown that treatment with Mangifera indica extract leads to a decrease in alloxan-induced glucose, urea, uric acid, and creatinine levels. A significant decrease in total protein, hemoglobin, body weight, albumin, and globulin were observed. Mangifera indica fed to diabetic rats reduced the effect of alloxan.

El-Gied et al. (2012) have studied the anti-microbial property of mango extracts. Doughari et al. (2008) found that the extract of
the leaf is effective against Staphylococcus aureus, Streptococcus pyogenase, Streptococcus pneumoniae, Bacillus cereus, Escherichia coli, Pseudomonas aerugenosa, Proteus mirabilis, Salmonella typhi, and Shigella flexnerr.

Olorunfemi et al. (2012) studied the anti-inflammatory and anti-pyretic impact of leaf extracts of mango on wistar rats. They concluded that mango extracts have significant analgesic effects on rats. Jiang et al, 2012. studied rats for the effect of mango extract as an anti-gout agent, and the results showed that there was considerable potential. The anti-ulcer property of the leaves of mango has been demonstrated in studies conducted by Neelima et al. (2012). Mango stem bark extracts were seen to be a useful anti-venom medicine against Russel viper's poison (Dhananjaya et al., 2011).

The fruit pulp has been demonstrated to have significant immunostimulant potential in mice (Naved et al., 2005). Garcia-Rivera et al. (2011) studied and validated the anti-tumor property of mango bark against breast cancer cells. Joona et al. (2013) studied the action of some natural products prepared from mango leaves to conclude that the leaves have potential for therapeutic use in cancer treatment.

Photochemical analysis of the composition of the extract has isolated a range of alkaloids, anthraquinones, reducing sugars, flavonoids, glycosides, saponins, cardiac glycosides, steroids, and tannins.

Mango Butter

Mango butter is extracted from the seed kernel through the solvent extraction process. The oil content of butter lies between 8-10%. The oil has a soft yellow color and melts at a range of 32-42 degrees Celsius. The butter stays in a semi-solid state at room temperature, melting on contact with the skin. The butter is rich in Palmitic and Stearic acids with content of the former compound being 16-18% and the latter 24-29%.

These properties make the butter suitable for use in moisturizing, anti-aging, anti-wrinkle, and skincare products. Many nature-based skin product manufacturers use mango butter in their formulations. The butter has a composition and properties like cocoa and shea butter. This makes mango butter a useful substitute for either of those.

Kittiphoom et al. (2013) conducted experiments that show that the oil from the kernel is a good source of the unsaturated fatty acid and phenolic compounds. These have potential for use in manufacture of nutrient-rich food oil and as ingredients for functional or enriched foods.

Mango wood is used in furniture making, construction, preparing veneers, and packing material. Mango wood is moderately strong and lies between the two extremes of hardwood and softwood.

Azadirachta indica – the natural antibiotic

Azadirachta indica probably has its origin in the Indian subcontinent. However, efforts to ascribe a single origin to a species may not stand scientific scrutiny because most species evolved over broad and similar ecosystems across the planet.

Azadirachta indica grows in the dry deciduous areas of more than 50 tropical countries across the world. Neem was introduced a century ago, first in Africa, and then, Latin America. The tree can grow up to 20 meters in height.

In the Asia Pacific and the African regions, neem is regarded an invasive species. In South Asia, it is observed to thrive in semi-arid ecological zones. The leaves of the branches are good fodder for goats, sheep, and even cattle. Palatability of neem to cattle, goats, and sheep makes the species highly susceptible to biotic damage both from wild and domesticated grazing animals.

It is famous for its medicinal properties. The earliest archaeological reference available on neem is seen on pottery from the Indus Valley Civilization (2600-1800 BC) period. An amulet recovered from Chanu Dora in Harappa, now in Pakistan, shows a man kneeling before what looks like a neem tree.

According to Hindu mythology, the oceans were churned by the gods and demons together until a pot of nectar of immortality (amrit) emerges from the depth of the mythical ocean. A fight ensues between the two sides to secure this pot. In this jostling, a drop of nectar spilled over from the pot and dropped onto earth. The neem tree emerged at that place. (I notice a similarity between this story and the Greek tale describing the mythical origin of the olive.) The neem is one of the ten trees in the nandanavana (Nandan Forest) of Ramayana.[18]

---

18   Ramayana epic origin is shrouded in mystery. The central character, Rama, in this epic, is said to be born in c. 3150 BC (Srinivasan, 2015).

Neem is valued for its medicinal properties. In Sanskrit, neem is called "arista," meaning "perfect, complete, and imperishable." It is also referred as "nimbati systhyadadati," i.e., "giver of good health," and as "Pinchumada," or "destroyer of leprosy and healer of skin infections." In Ayurveda, the tree is regarded as a "sarva roga nivarni," i.e., a "universal reliever of all illness."

The tree is also referred to as "Sitala mata" tree, which would roughly translate to "mother with cooling property." Neem is called "Shajar-e-Munarak," or the "blessed tree" by Unani scholars. The Persians called it "Azad dirakht-i-Hind," or "the noble tree of India."

In Medicine

The tree is mentioned in the Susrutasamhita and the Charakasamhita (dated in the 1st millennium BC). Kautilya, also called Chanakya, the famous statesman and political thinker from the 4th century BC, also mentions neem in his seminal work Arthasastra.

Emperor Ashoka (3rd century BC) is said to have ordered that neem trees be planted in every village in his vast dominions encompassing the whole of South Asia—from modern day Afghanistan down to peninsular South India. The Brihat Samhita, the encyclopedia work of Varahmahira composed in the 6thcentury AD, enunciates the medicinal properties of the tree. He too recommends planting the tree in all villages.

Small pox and chicken pox were treated by the plant. The skin of people affected was brushed lightly with a branch of the tree, to drive "evil spirits" away. A disinfecting bath with neem leaves was also recommended.

Symbolic chewing of the bitter neem leaves followed by eating sweets is a New Year celebration ritual in many communities. Many regions in India have spring-based New Year festivals like Ugadi, Pongal, etc. The dates of these regional New Year festivities vary from region to region.

It is widely believed by people that the presence of a neem tree near

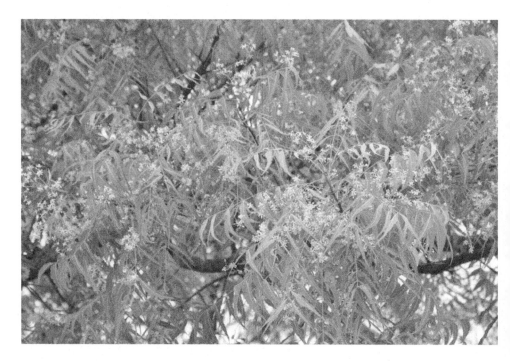

Picture 13 Azadirachta indica in bloom
Photo: Dr Ravikumar, Senior Botanist, FRLHT

dwellings helps improve human health. Other traditional medicinal uses of the tree include its use as a natural contraceptive. The anti-septic property of neem leaf extracts has traditionally been used to check the growth of pimples and acne, but this myth was busted when a study concluded that the species does not possess anti-acne properties (Nand et al., 2012). Drinking neem juice first thing in the morning is said to be effective in treating a urinary tract infection.

The tree acts as a prophylactic against multiple infectious diseases like malaria, cholera, diarrhea, etc. The tree is said to be a purifier of air. The bark of the tree is ground in the form of a paste and applied to heal boils and wounds. Neem has been shown to boost immunity, help purify blood, and act as a detoxifier. Numerous Ayurvedic medicines containing neem have been manufactured and these are sold in the Indian market.

The ripe fruit is sweet and helps keep the body free of infections. Its diverse medicinal properties have led to the tree being christened "The Village Pharmacy." The tree has a place in the Indian Pharmacopeia.

Neem is one of the most researched trees worldwide with over 2,000 clinical trials and studies. A wide range of its traditional medicinal properties have been validated through animal trials, including the anti-helminthic, anti-fungal, antibacterial, antiviral, anti-diabetic, antioxidant, anti-cancer, anti-malarial, wound healing, contraceptive, spermicidal, and sedative properties.

The plant is used to treat a range of skin diseases like scabies, leprosy, and skin ulcers. It is also used to treat eye disorders, a bloody nose, an upset stomach, loss of appetite, cardiovascular issues, intestinal issues, fever, gum, malaria, etc. The fruit helps treat hemorrhoids, urinary tract disorders, intestinal worms, and provides relief in headaches. It is regarded as a mosquito repellent and a diuretic.

Neem contains 40 different active compounds called limonoids. The main active ingredient of neem seed is Azadirachtin. The active ingredients isolated from neem include a variety of saponins, triterpenoids, flavonoids, and a range of alkaloids and tannin. Some of the popular molecules isolated from the tree are Nimbin, Nimbidin, Nimbidol, Gedunin, Sodium Nimbinate, Quercetin, Salannin, and Azadirachtin. Each of these molecules is responsible for one or more medicinal properties of the plant, as elaborated below:

1. Nimbin: anti-inflammatory, anti-pyretic, anti-histamine, anti-fungal
2. Nimbidin: antibacterial, anti-ulcer, analgesic, anti-arrhythmic, anti-fungal
3. Ninbidol: anti-tubercular, anti-protozoal, anti-pyretic
4. Gedunin: vasodilator, anti-malaria, anti-fungal
5. Sodium nimbinate: diuretic, spermicide, anti-arthritic
6. Quercetin: anti-protozoal
7. Salannin: insect repellent
8. Azadirchtin: insect repellent, anti-feedant, anti-hormonal

The anti-malarial potential of the plant has been studied by many scientists. Preliminary results indicate that the species can be used in vector control (Awofeso, 2011; Bedri et al., 2013; and Habluetzel et al., 2009). Experiments for Alzheimer's disease control conducted on rats have shown positive results (Raghavendra et al., 2013).

The study by Asif et al. (2013) shows that the species possesses spermicidal potential. Similar properties were observed in a study conducted on albino rats (Aladakatti et al., 2006). The study by Khan et al. (2013) indicates that the plant has immunomodulatory and anti-cancerous properties.

Experiments on rats with induced hepatotoxicity and genotoxicity proved its chemoprotective effects (Singh et al., 2012). A fractionated neem-leaf extract sold under the name IRAB/IRACARP in Nigeria is reported to be effective against malaria, HIV/AIDS, and cancer (Anyaehie, 2009).

Antimicrobial Properties

The level of anti-microbial activities of the A. indica oil depends on both the protein and carbohydrate contents. The higher the level of protein and carbohydrate content in the extract, the better is the observed anti-microbial activity (Asif, 2012). The anti-microbial property of the plant has been studied and reported extensively (Grover et al., 2011; Khan et al., 2010; and Bharitkar et al., 2013).

The anti-fungal property against the candida class of fungi was observed in experiments by Llyod et al. (2005) and against Schistocerca gregaria by Sharma et al. (2008). This property was also observed against fungi of the Fusarium genus (Geraldo et al., 2010). The plant has nematocidal potential too (Akhtar, 2000).

Antidiabetic Action

Azadirachta indica leaf extract and seed oil, when administered in normal as well as diabetic rabbits, was observed to have a hypoglycemic effect comparable to the anti-diabetic medicine glibenclamide. It can be safely deduced that A. indica could benefit diabetes mellitus patients. It was helpful in preventing or delaying the onset of the disease (Khosla et al., 2000).

The antidiabetic potential of quercetin molecule found in the leaves of the plant was studied and antidiabetic potential of the molecule observed (Chourasiya et al., 2012). The species was seen to prevent the onset of long-term deleterious effects from diabetes (Shailey et al., 2012).

Studies on mice have confirmed the ethno-medical use of neem leaf extracts as potential hepato-protective agents (Kalaivani et al., 2009).

Industrial and Agricultural Use

Oil is extracted from the seed and can be used as a lubricant. Neem cake, a by-product of neem oil extraction, is a natural fertilizer. The cake, when ploughed into the soil, protects plant roots from nematodes and white ants. The oil is an increasingly popular organic insecticide and pesticide. With the organic movement rising in popularity across the globe, neem has the potential to displace traditional chemical insecticides and pesticides in use today.

Neem oil is not an instantly effective insecticide. Spraying it on crops does not result in the immediate elimination of harmful insects and pests. The action of the oil on the pests and insects is through their hormone system, with their metabolism being affected. Insects, on ingesting the oil, stop eating and are unable to breed, propagate, and proliferate, breaking their lifecycle. In time, the pests die, and the entire colony disappears. Pest eggs are also not able to hatch, and the larvae are not able to molt.

Chewing and sucking insects only get impacted by neem oil. The action of neem is selective with destruction restricted to only this variety of pests. Neem oil acts slowly, unlike the fast-acting chemical insecticides, but the action is long lasting. The quantities of neem oil required are also much smaller, and the insecticide action takes place at very low concentrations.

Neem oil is a very powerful anti-feedant and insect repellent. The oil is especially susceptible to ultraviolet light. As it is a systemic insecticide, the oil in the diluted form can be applied to the soil from where it is taken up by the plants. The insecticidal action takes place in-situ. An insect may take a bite or two of such plants but then stop, due to systemic impact.

Azadirachtin forms 90% of neem oil insecticide. Salannin, another substance obtained from neem, is a powerful repellent deterring pest
from biting on plants that otherwise they would love to feed upon. The deterrent action is stated to be more powerful than the synthetic chemical called "Deet" (N N Diethyl meta toluamide). Deet is an ingredient in most of the insect repellents commonly found in the market.

The biopesticide action of neem commences when an insect larva feeds on the plant, when the active molecules in neem—azadirachtin, salanin, and melandriol—cause an anti-peristalitic wave in the alimentary canal in the insect, causing a vomiting sensation that forces them to stop feeding.

Neem also prevents the female from depositing eggs on the plant (Lokanandan et al., 2012). Various analyses have validated the natural insecticidal property of neem leaves (Boadu et al., 2011; Siddiquia et al., 2004; Satti et al., 2013; Nicoletti et al, 2010.; and Schmutterer, 1990).

Mixed results were obtained when the effect of neem in counteracting the negative effect on plants suffering from fungus infestation was studied as the extract was effective against some fungi and not against others (Hazmi, 2013).

Neem oil is also useful against fungi, mildew, and rust. Pure oil is colored and cloudy with a sulfurous, nutty, garlic smell. It solidifies at low temperature and requires to be warmed before application.

Neem Cake

Neem cake is used as an organic manure and is a by-product of the oil extraction process. The oil is produced by cold pressing neem seeds. The high Azadirachtin content in neem cake helps protect crops against parasitic nematodes and pests, and acts as soil conditioner.

The anti-feedant, insecticidal chemicals in the cake like azadirachtin, salannin, nimbin, and azadiradione make the cake not just as an organic fertilizer but also a natural soil insecticide and fungicide.

Neem cake is constituted of nitrogen, (2-5%), phosphorus (0.5-1%), potassium (1-2%), calcium (0.5-3%), magnesium (0.3-1%), sulfur (0.2-3%), zinc (15-60 ppm), copper (4-20 ppm), iron (5001,200 ppm),
and manganese (20-60 ppm). It is rich in both sulfur compounds and bitter limonoids.[19]

An infusion of neem seed powder in water makes for an organic insecticide. Crushed dried leaves are put in cupboards and grain storage bins to keep insects and pests away. Gum that occasionally exudes from the tree is used as a demulcent tonic. The blossoms of the plant are used in a variety of culinary preparations.

Production

Exports of neem-based products by India in 2012 was valued at US $5.73 million. This includes neem seeds which formed 2.79% of the total exports of neem products by value (EXIM Bank, Iyer. The US and Italy are the leading importers of neem extracts from India. With $2.62 million imports in 2011-12, the US was the largest importer of neem extracts from India, followed by Japan and Spain. Japan was the largest importer of neem oil cakes from India, valued at $0.28 million in 2011-12.

---

19   (https://en.wikipedia.org/wiki/Neem_cake)

According to the estimates of Neem Foundation (a voluntary, independent, and non-profit organization), there are about 20 million neem trees in India (EXIM Bank Report, 2011).

Industry estimates say that neem trees in India bear 3.5 million metric tons of kernel every year. These can yield around 700,000 metric tons of neem oil. Most of the neem production in India is for use within the country.

In Oral Care

Neem was tested for its effectiveness against different infectious microorganisms (Gram positive bacteria and Gram-negative bacteria), such as bacterial strains of S. aureus, E. coli, B. cerus, P. vulgaris, S. typhi, K. pneumoniae, and S. dysenteriae, and fungal strains of F. oxysporum, A. flavus, A. fumigates, A. niger, C. albicans, Cladosporium sp., M. canis, M. gypseum, T. rubrum, T. mentagrophytes, P. notatum, P. citrinum, etc. (Prashant et al., 2007; and Sorna et al., 2011).

Neem was studied for its anti-gingivitis and anti-plaque properties and as a mouth rinse. The results showed it to be an effective dental and oral anti-septic agent (Chatterjee et al., 2011; Kaushik et al., 2012; Marco et al., 2008; and Nayak et al., 1979).

All parts of the tree from the fruit, leaves, branches, and bark are used. Twigs of neem are used as natural toothbrush; the anti-septic action of the plant keeps the mouth clean and hygienic. Toothpaste with neem extracts is sold extensively in India.

Neem is said to destroy bacteria causing pyorrhea and gingivitis—the two most common of the gum diseases. It prevents cell adhesion and helps to control plaque. Chatterjee et al. (2011) have demonstrated a significant reduction of gingival, bleeding, and plaque formation in patient trials conducted over a period of 21 days using neem extracts. The results obtained were compared with a placebo set.

Extracts from neem sticks or bark are shown to inhibit the growth of Streptococcus mutans. Significant reductions in bacterial adhesion in-vitro suggests that the plant can reduce the damage caused by streptococci bacteriaon the surface of the tooth. Neem extract produced the maximum zone of inhibition on Streptococcus mutans at 50% concentration.

Other Streptococcus species which are involved in the development of dental caries such as Streptococcus salivarius, Streptococcus mitis, and Streptococcus sanguis are also inhibited by neem extracts (Prashant et al., 2007). The antibacterial activity of the aqueous extract of neem on Lactobacillus sp has also been noticed at higher concentrations of neem (Sorna et al., 2011). Various studies have demonstrated that neem-based mouth rinses are highly efficacious and are emerging as an alternative therapy in the treatment of periodontal diseases.

In Skin Care and Cosmetics

Neem oil is used to make hair healthy, improve liver function, detoxify the blood, and balance blood-sugar levels. It is rich in long-chain fatty acids, causing the oil to be rapidly absorbed into the skin. The oil is used in skin moisturizers.

Oil is used in cosmetics, soaps, shampoos, balms, creams, and toothpaste. Many these manufactured products are sold in stores across India. Bathing in neem water keeps the skin healthy and relieves skin ailments. Neem is also used in face and hair packs. Neem oil is believed to slow down graying of hair.

CHAPTER IV

Spices from India

There were three major civilizations—Egypt, Mesopotamia, and Indus Valley—in the chalcolithic period (copper age). Harappan seals and ceramic ware with Indus valley markings have been recovered from Susa and Ur (Kramer, 1964). These were two major cities of ancient Mesopotamia. Ur was one of the earliest towns of Sumer. This city existed in the Euphrates River region of modern-day Iraq.

Indus Valley Civilization was the largest of the three ancient civilizations covering an area of 1.25 million km. The analysis of tooth enamel from human remains found buried at Harappa indicate that some residents came from foreign lands like Mesopotamia and neighboring regions.

Archaeological excavations at Mehrgah in Baluchistan, Pakistan, reveal that settled life in the Indian subcontinent began around 7500 BC (Jarrige et al., 1995). This society slowly evolved over the millennia into a well-planned urban civilization called Indus Valley Civilization, or the Harappan Civilization. Harappan Civilization is divided into three distinct stages: Early Harappan (3300-2600 BC), Mature Harappan (2600-2000 BC), and Late Harappan (2000-1700 BC).

These people lived in modern urban centers with streets, drains, water tanks, etc. arranged in a symmetrical layout. Some historians suggest that the Indus Valley Civilization people were of Dravidian stock, ancestors of the Dravidians who inhabit the southern peninsular region of India today. This theory considers all South Asia, including Afghanistan, to have been inhabited by Dravidians.

Unfortunately, the script of this civilization has not yet been deciphered, and our understanding is limited to the interpretation and analysis of archaeological findings. Many of the seals found from the Indus cities bear figures of animals like the unicorn and the deer. Some depict the flora, like the leaf of peepal, a species of Ficus sps that is revered by Hindus to this day.

Images of a variety of animals like elephant, rhinoceros, deer, etc. indicate the existence of a moister and wetter habitat with a less arid climate than that which exists today. All the major sites lie along the Indus and its tributaries, all which flow into the Arabian Sea after crisscrossing the Northwestern region of the subcontinent.

Whole cities have been excavated in Harappa and Mohenjo-Daro, and these sites are in the Punjab and Sindh regions of Pakistan today. Trade caravans were known to ply between the Indus Valley through modern day Afghanistan to distant lands of Iran and Iraq. Sargon, the famous Mesopotamian King (who lived around 2234-2279 BC) had scribes who kept written records of foreign ships visiting his territory. From these records, we learn that gold, copper, and jewelry was imported from Meluha.[20]

Plank-based boats with single mast and sail were said to have been in use in this period. To reach Mesopotamia by boat, vessels had to keep close to the coast. The entire coastline from India to Mesopotamia was dotted with small ports, and at each port, provisions would be taken onboard. Lothal, the prominent port city, lay on the Sabarmati River in present day Gujarat.

For a journey to Egypt, boats would cross the narrow Straits of Hormuz. Once across, they would stick to the coastal waters onto their onwards voyage to the Red Sea. These were perilous journeys carried out by intrepid ancient traders and mariners. Middlemen merchants from Dilmun (Bahrain of today), an intermediate location en route from India to Egypt and Greece, were part of this complex trail of logistics.

---

20   "Meluha" means "dark people." This information is used to support the theory that the Indus Valley Civilization and the region beyond it in the Indian Peninsula was inhabited by Dravidians. Dravidians have darker skin and now inhabit southern parts of India.

Storage jars and pottery from the Indus Valley have been recovered from the beaches of Oman. An account of Pericles from 1st century AD records honey, spices, and ghee (clarified butter) amongst a long list of products that were traded from India to the dominions of Rome.

Many popular spices like pepper and cinnamon and timber like sandalwood, teak, etc. were imported from India into Greece, Rome, and Egypt. Cotton was grown extensively, and the Indus Valley was one of its major exporters to Mesopotamia and Egypt.

Food in the Indus Valley

Discoveries by Kashyap et al., 2011 indicate that spices and herbs in use then were not different to those in use today. Examining human teeth and the residue from cooking pots, Kashyap spotted telltale signs of turmeric and ginger. A carbonized clove of garlic has been found in excavations done at the burial site, dated between 2500 and 2200 BC, located at Farmana in Haryana.

McIntosh's research on the Harappans revealed that people ate a variety of fruit, vegetables, and spices. This includes a variety of brassica, brown mustard greens, coriander, dates, jujube, walnuts, grapes, figs, mango, okra, caper, sugarcane, garlic, turmeric, ginger, cumin, and cinnamon. These may have been either cultivated locally or gathered from the wild. Sesame and linseed were cultivated to obtain edible oil (McIntosh, 2008).

Incense and Beauty Care

Incense cisterns have been recovered from the Indus Valley sites, but there is no concrete scientific evidence pointing us toward the type of plants used as incense. We are left to speculate based on the archeological finds unearthed from that period.

From this, we can deduce that traditional herbs, spices, cosmetics, and incense in use today in India were also used 5,000-6,000 years ago. Ecological changes over the millennia may have made some parts of the region unsuited for some herbs and plants, but from an evolutionary standpoint, 6,000 years is but a moment of time.

Commencement of the Vedic Period

The Indus Civilization went into decline around the middle of the 2nd millennium BC. The decline was probably a consequence of rapid change in the local ecology. Saraswati, a major river that flowed through Northwest India, disappeared probably from a tectonic event causing a rapid desertification of a hitherto fertile region.

The immediate cause of this decline could be a flooding of the Indus Valley. This displacement and the subsequent desertification would have led to impoverishment of the society. People would have been forced to migrate out of the region.

There is also a popular hypothesis that the people of the Indus Valley were ousted by a more mobile fighting race of people who came from Central Asia to India. These were the Aryans who currently inhabit most of the Northern India. The theories on the origin of Aryans are hotly debated by historians. Some believe that the Aryans migrated from Central Asia to India, while others contest this with the claim that Aryans are of Indian origin.

Be that is it may, it is widely accepted that the foundation of the Hindu religion is based on four Vedas and the six Vedangas, which are products of the Aryan age. Additional ancient Hindu literature also includes Meemamsa or interpretations, Nyaya (logic), Puranas, and Shastras.

The gods of the Vedic age, their food, herbs, spices, and medicine all originate in nature, as is the case with other ancient societies.

Ancient Evidence on Spices

It was only when the Mauryan Empire came into existence (320-185 BC) that records of formal interaction between the Greeks and Indian rulers became available to us. Greeks were prolific writers who recorded their experiences in writing, giving us a wealth of material to understand this era. This is supplemented with archaeological evidence, inscriptions, and in later years, writings on the palm leaf discovered from various parts of India and China. Written evidence of ancient Indian practices, though, is limited. Transmission of knowledge from generation to generation in ancient India was largely oral.

Megasthenes was an ambassador sent by Seleucus (302-291 BC) to the court of the first of the Mauryan Kings—Chandragupta. He visited the valley of the Ganges River, which has remained the most populated region of the subcontinent. Megasthenes mentions spices being brought to the Ganges River from the southern parts of India. Apparently, there existed a vibrant trade in spices between various parts of the subcontinent.

The spices mentioned by Megasthenes were coriander, cumin, asafetida, cloves, and indigenous spices like pepper, turmeric, sesame, and mustard. Asafetida would have been an import from Afghanistan and Iran. Cloves, perhaps, came from the Indonesian Islands and Africa. Cumin and coriander were, most probably, imports too. Today, most of these spices are grown in India.

The ports along the Arabian Sea have been in existence at least as far back as the 2nd millennium BC. Lothal, the port on the Sabarmati River in Gujarat, was in existence from at least 2400 BC. Berthing facilities for ships have been excavated there. An active trade with the Assyrians, Sumerians, and Mesopotamians took place through this port. The route across the Arabian Sea that aided ships to travel fast on the back of monsoon wind currents had not yet been discovered.

Spices from South India

From the 4th century BC onwards, pepper and cardamom, along with areca nut, have been cultivated in the evergreen and semi-evergreen monsoonal regions of the India's southern region. These commodities were exported from ports that dotted both on the east and west coast of peninsular India.

Muziris was one such major port, near the modern port and naval base of Kochi, Kerala. It was an important export hub for goods destined for Greece and Rome. With the Romans establishing their dominance over territory on both sides of the Red Sea, an unimpeded flow of goods from India to the region took place.

Trade from Muziris to the Red Sea region flourished from the 2nd century AD to the middle of the first millennium. The Roman port at Alexandria in Egypt became the clearing house port at the far end of the Red Sea. At its peak, the Romans are believed to have sent around 120 ships a year from Egypt to Muziris.

Exports from India included, among other commodities, vast quantities of pepper. Pliny estimates that a million sesterii worth of goods was imported from the southwestern coast ports of India to Rome. By then, the hereto undiscovered sea route based on the monsoon winds was used to make the voyage between the two regions much quicker. Trade between India and Rome flourished during this period, references to which are made in the records kept in Periplus Maris Erythraei in the 1st century AD.

India was not a single unified kingdom for long periods of time in its history. Even in the Mauryan period, the southernmost region of the Indian subcontinent was ruled by independent kings, outside the direct rule of the emperor. The capital of the Mauryan Empire was Pataliputra, in modern day Patna, the capital of the eastern state of Bihar.

However, the Mauryan dominions stretched to the far west, encompassing land up to modern Afghanistan. In the east, the empire control extended to the eastern part of the South Asian peninsular seaboard and included today's Myanmar.

The ports on the Bay of Bengal were transshipment ports for ships bringing goods from the Indonesian Islands for sale within India and for re-export to the Persian Gulf and the Red Sea region. Some of the major transshipment ports on the eastern seaboard included Tamralipti, Palur, Kalingapatnam, Arikamedu, Poompuhar, etc. Spices and other commodities were traded through these ports.

Indian cuisine is famous for its extensive use of spices. However, India has never been a monolith in culture, language, and tradition. The same is true for its cuisine. There are, however, some common fundamental principles of food common to all South Asia. Indian food is categorized into six tastes: sweet, sour, salty, spicy, bitter, and astringent. A well-balanced Indian meal should contain all six tastes.

As in other ancient societies from the Biblical region to India, herbs and spices were used in flavoring, as preservative, for nutrition as well as medicine. Some of the common traditional local spices included turmeric, cloves, cardamoms, ginger, etc.

Turmeric (Curcuma longa) – a spice with multiple medicinal properties

Turmeric plant is a perennial herbaceous plant from the ginger family. Turmeric is the boiled and dried rhizome of this plant. Propagation of the species is done vegetative, with rhizomes. It is native to India, Japan, Korea, China, East and West Africa, South Pacific Islands, Carribbean Islands, and Central America.

Turmeric rhizomes are ground to yield a deep orange-yellow colored powder. The spice has a distinct earthy with slightly bitter, peppery flavor. The spice has been in use in India since the earliest of times, as we know from the analysis of pots from the Indus Valley Civilization. (Weber et al, 2011).

There existed an extensive trade with the Assyrians, Mesopotamians, and Persians with India since the time of the Indus Valley Civilization. Ancient tablets of Ashurbanipal (7th century BC) have listed large numbers of aromatic spices that were in use in the region, one that includes turmeric. Turmeric was probably used both in cuisine and as medicine. King Merodach-baladan II (721-710 BC) kept records of the different species of plants, including herbs and spices that were cultivated in his garden (Tapsell, 2006).

It finds mention in the Ebers Papyrus (c. 1500 BC) from Egypt where, as in India, it was used in cleaning wounds and as an anti-septic. The spice was mixed with honey to prepare an external ointment. In India, turmeric and clarified butter are heated and the ointment used to treat wounds. Turmeric enhances circulation in the affected region and aids the healing process.

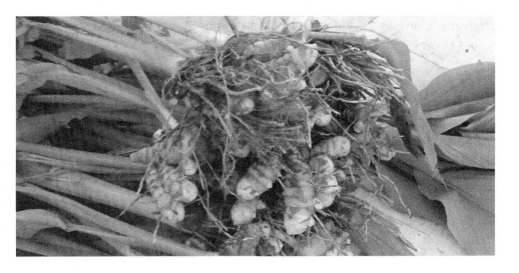

Picture 14 Curcuma longa (turmeric)
Photo: Sudhir Ahluwalia

Hindus regard turmeric as highly auspicious. The Mahabharata refers to the application of turmeric to purify the body. The tradition of applying turmeric paste on both the groom and the bride continues to this day in Hindu weddings in certain parts of India

Dioscorides, too, lists turmeric as a medicinal remedy. He refers to it as a yellow spice. He relates the spice to ginger. Theophrastus, (317-287 BC) in his writings, calls it an aromatic spice, "khroma," meaning "color" in Greek. The Roman Emperor Diocletian (284-305 AD) mentions use of what he refers to as the Arabian saffron, probably because turmeric was supplied to the Roman army by Arabian merchants. Arabian traders brought turmeric to the region from India.

Turmeric, however, makes for a poor fabric dye as its color fades quickly. It was used by ancient Buddhist monks to dye their robes and saris. Hindu saints, too, wear turmeric yellow robes. In Hindu spiritualism, the orange-yellow color is regarded as a mark of spirituality and renunciation. Yellow is also regarded as a color of sacrifice. Warriors from kingdoms in the Western Indian region, which today is constituted into the state of Rajasthan, would don yellow head scarves when entering a do-or-die battle.

Traditionally, the yellow-colored spice is associated with the sun as it is the color of the solar plexus chakra[21] associated with the metabolic and digestive systems. It is also the color of the sacral chakra associated with the reproductive system.

In Food

It is a food additive and is used to color cheese, yoghurt, salad dressings, butter, and as a spice in curries. Turmeric is used extensively in the Middle East, Persia and Southeast Asia. It gives food not just a distinct yellow color but a unique flavor too. Turmeric leaves, when wrapped around cooked food, give it a distinct flavor.

---

21   According to the Siddha system of medicine, chakras are regarded as centers of energy in the human body. The body is said to have seven chakras.

Turmeric is a food preservative added to the Indian pickle. Mixed with oil, the two helps preserve the fruit. It extends the shelf life of cottage cheese to up to 2 weeks.

In Skin Care

Turmeric is used extensively in cosmetics and skincare products. Several turmeric-based skincare products like creams, body scrubs, anti-aging, anti-wrinkle formulations, etc. are sold in stores across South Asia and the Middle East. Turmeric gives the skin softness and glow. Saraf et al. (2011) studied and validated the anti-aging, anti-wrinkle action of a cosmetic cream with Curcuma longa.

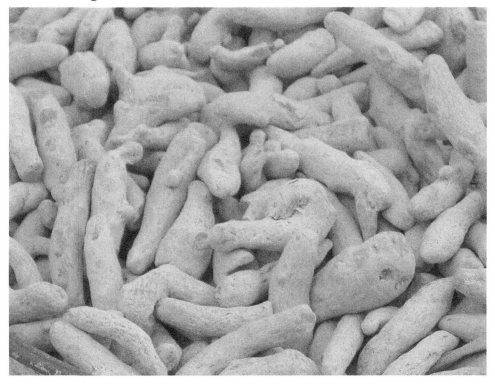

Picture 15 Turmeric spice
Photo: Dr Ravikumar, Senior botanist, FRLHT

Turmeric is an excellent pesticide too. Sprinkling turmeric powder water near the entry points of your house is said to keep insects, ants, and termites away.

In Medicine

Traditionally, it has been used to treat skin, gastrointestinal, autoimmune, liver, eye, and other disorders. Turmeric is said to provide relief in allergies, gall bladder ailments, edema, tumors, and cataract. Its anti-inflammatory and antibacterial properties are used to treat inflammations and infections.

Curcumin is the yellow pigment in turmeric and has been in use as medicine for centuries. Curcuminoides have been extracted from turmeric (Kulkarni et al., 2012) Pharmacological reviews undertaken by Ammon et al. (1991), Jurenka (2009), and others validate curcumin's anti-inflammatory property. Curcumin, the active compound in the spice, exhibits anti-spasmodic activity. It was seen to stimulate bile secretion in animals and help treat liver disorders.

Araujo et al. (2001) and Aggarwal et al. (2007 and 2009) have noted the anti-cancer, antiviral, antibacterial, anti-fungal, and gastrointestinal actions of curcumin. It is also helpful in treating liver and other ailments. Curcumin is said to prevent Alzheimer's disease (Balasubramanian, 2006; Yanagisawa et al., 2010; Yang et al., 2004; Lee 2002; and Tomiyama, 2010).

The action of turmeric oil molecule ar-tumerone was studied by Jankasem et al. (2013), and its anti-fungal property on skin was validated. The anti-microbial property of turmeric was observed in experiments conducted by Khan et al. in 2009.

Curcuma longa is a lesser-known drug in homoeopathy. Even then, its traditionally accepted medicinal properties were subjected to a multicentric clinical trial. Turmeric was found to be useful in treating anxiety, dementia, dysmenorrhea, gingivitis, toothache, lumbago, pharyngitis, etc. (Chakraborty et al., 2011).

A study conducted by Kim et al. (2009) validated the impact of turmeric in checking the replication of the hepatitis B virus. The hepatoprotective effect of the species was observed in rats induced with liver cirrhosis (Salama et al., 2013). The antioxidant activity of the species was observed in experiments by Yadav et al. (2013).

The insect repellent action of ar-tumerone and tumerone was validated in a study conducted by Su et al. (1982). Nephrotoxicity in rats caused by mercury-based compounds was observed to ameliorate with turmeric extract and curcumin, showing bright of its use in treating cases of mercury poisoning affecting the kidney (Joshi et al., 2013).

Turmeric was shown to prevent fetus implantation in the uterus of rats. This holds out the prospect of its use in fertility control (Yadav et al., 2011). Anti-cancer properties of turmeric have also been reported (Basnet et al, 2011)

The chemical composition of turmeric has been studied. The most important chemical components of turmeric are a group of compounds called curcuminoids, which include curcumin (diferuloylmethane), demethoxycurcumin, and bisdemethoxycurcumin. Curcumin constitutes 3.14% (on average) of powdered turmeric and gives the spice its peppery taste.

Curcumin is poorly absorbed into the bloodstream. Black pepper substantially enhances the absorption of curcumin. Ayurvedic physicians and nutritionists recommend mixing a pinch of turmeric in milk to be consumed at bedtime. This is said to help build immunity and is beneficial against multiple other ailments.

Jagetia and Aggarwal at the Department of Experimental Therapeutics, The University of Texas M. D. Anderson Cancer Center, Houston, US, writes, "Interestingly, curcumin at low doses can also enhance antibody responses. This suggests that curcumin's reported beneficial effects in arthritis, allergy, asthma, atherosclerosis, heart disease, Alzheimer's disease, diabetes, and cancer might be due in part to its ability to modulate the immune system."

Curcumin boosts levels of BDNF (brain derived neurotrophic factor), a protein and brain hormone which increases the growth of new neurons and fights various degenerative processes in the brain. Curcumin has beneficial effects against several factors known to play a role in heart disease.

Researchers from Cancer Biology Research Center, South Dakota, claim that curcumin may be an effective chemo-preventive and therapeutic agent for cervical cancer prevention and treatment. They found that curcumin treatment suppresses growth in cervical cancer cells by altering the HPV[22]-associated molecular pathways. Basic research appears to validate the ability of curcumin to suppress several stages of cancer.

It is believed to have the potential for treating Alzheimer's diseases, arthritis, and chronic illnesses. Stage 2, and in some cases, stage 3 clinical trials are underway to validate the anti-inflammatory, anti-cancer, and anti-Alzheimer's properties of turmeric (Cole et al., 2007).

Other properties of turmeric validated in trials include anti-spasmodic, nematocidal, chemo-protective, anti-HIV, anti-yeast, etc.

Studies by Drew Tortoriello, an endocrinologist and research scientist at the Naomi Berrie Diabetes Center at Columbia University Medical Center indicate that turmeric lessens insulin resistance and prevents type-2 diabetes. Curcumin, however, is not readily bio-available. Even those who are not pre-diabetic will benefit from regularly adding turmeric powder to their food.

Turmeric is water soluble and contains oxalates. It thins the blood, and so, is contraindicated with aspirin and warfarin. It is placed in the "generally recognized as safe" category of food additives by the FDA.

---

22   HPV, or the Human Papilloma Virus, according to CDC (Center for Disease Control and Prevention) is the most common sexually transmitted virus infection. In some cases, it is shown to cause cancer.

Production

India is the largest producer, consumer, and exporter of turmeric in the world. India accounts for about 80% of the global turmeric production. Other major producing areas include China, and several Central American and South East Asian countries. India's share of exports in global trade is around 60%.

Global production of turmeric is estimated to be around 1.1 million metric tons per annum. Asia consumes a lot of what it produces. UAE, Arab world, US, South Africa, Japan, Southeast Asian countries, and some European countries like the UK and Netherlands are the major importers of turmeric.

PEPPER – Indian spice exchanged for gold

There are two species of pepper producing plants. The more popular pepper comes from Piper nigrum. This pepper is available in four variants: black, white, green, and red. Piper longum is the other species which, at one time, was the most prized of peppers in Ancient Rome. This demand has now been largely replaced by chilly. In India, Piper longum—also called pippali in trade—is an ingredient of the Indian curry masala (garam masala).

The dried berries of Piper nigrum is commonly used in South Asian homes. Piper nigrum is a perennial climbing shrub. Pepper requires a hot and humid climate and is extensively cultivated in the coastal areas near the Western Ghats in South India. It is also cultivated in Indonesia, Malaysia, Sri Lanka, Thailand, China, Vietnam, Cambodia, Brazil, Mexico, and Gautemala.

The pepper plant is an epiphyte, i.e., it requires support for climbing. In India, it is intercropped with areca nut and coconut. Pepper vines cling to the trunks of these trees. The pepper-yielding berry bunches are arranged in the form of an inflorescence. Abundant rain, moisture, rivers, and the water found in the Western Indian coastal region is ideal for this spice crop. Pepper continues, even today, to be one of the most important spice crops of India.

Pepper Type and Use in Food

Pepper is marketed in four different colors: black, white, red, and green. All four varieties are harvested from the same plant. This is done by altering the time of harvest and varying the method of processing.

To produce black pepper, the berries are picked when they begin turning yellow. Sun-drying these berries, plucked just before they are fully ripe, produces the black variety of pepper. At this stage the berries have an excellent flavor.

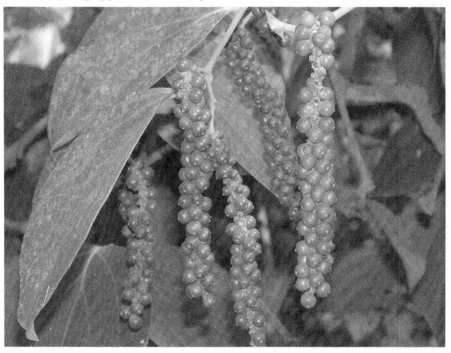

Picture 16 Piper nigrum fruit
Photo: Dr Ravikumar, Senior Botanist, FRLHT

The white pepper is picked when the berries are riper. The outer skin of the berry is removed to reveal the lighter colored pepper underneath. If berries are harvested early, pickled in salt or vinegar, and dried at high temperature, it yields green pepper. The unripe green pepper berries are highly aromatic and have an herbal flavor. Green pepper is less pungent. Red peppercorns are produced from ripe berries after pickling them in salt or vinegar and then drying them at a high temperature.

Pepper plants in Indonesia are grayish black in color, less aromatic, and produce smaller berries when compared to Indian pepper. Pepper from Malaysia is mild and fruity. Brazilian pepper is also very mild.

Pepper and long pepper have been extensively used in India since the earliest of times. Long pepper and black and white peppers are important ingredients of garam masala.[23] Spice ingredients are roasted and ground together to make curry/garam masala.

There are regional differences in the composition of masala in India. Curry masala is blended with herbs and ground to make a paste. The paste can be made with water, vinegar, coconut milk, nuts, onions, garlic, turmeric, etc. and used to flavor the curry. Coconut milk is not used in North Indian cuisine. Other ingredients like star anise, cubeb, etc. are also added at times, and the ratio of the various spices in the blend can be adjusted to taste.

A typical Indian version of curry masala contains the following spices:

1. Black and white peppercorns
2. Cloves
3. Cinnamon or cassia bark
4. Nutmeg and mace
5. Black and green cardamom pods
6. Tej patta or Indian bay leaf

23 Garam masala is the curry masala popular in South Asian cuisine.

Given the close trading and cultural ties between India and the Mediterranean, Persian, and Arabic worlds, it is not surprising that black pepper is an integral part of the Arabic spice baharat. Individual cuisines can have their own mixes with the key ingredients staying common.

A typical recipe for baharat is a mixture of the following finely ground ingredients:

- 4 parts black pepper
- 3 parts coriander seeds
- 3 parts cinnamon
- 3 parts cloves
- 4 parts cumin seeds
- 1 part cardamom pods
- 3 parts nutmeg
- 6 parts paprika

Historical Overview

We are aware that there existed a vibrant trading relation, primarily maritime, between the southern coast of India and Ancient Egypt. Arab traders in the Red Sea region played an important role as intermediaries to this trade.

The importance of the spice in ancient societies can be gauged from the fact that black peppercorns were found stuffed in the nostrils of the mummy of Ramesses II (c. 1213 BC) . It must have been a valuable commodity for it to be chosen for use on the Pharaoh's body.

With the Greek influence extending beyond Macedonia to Persia and Afghanistan, cultural interaction between India and Greece got a major boost. Both long and black pepper were imported by the Greeks and the Romans. It was a spice that was much sought after by the rich and famous of the time.

Hippocrates mentions the use of long pepper as a medicament. Theophrastus distinguished between the long pepper and black pepper. For some time, it was believed that the long and black peppers came from the same plant. This confusion on origins of long and black peppers continued up to the 1st century AD. Pliny, the Roman historian

and philosopher, believed that black pepper came from the same plant that produced long pepper.

Pliny the Elder's Natural History tells us that the price per pound of long pepper was 15 denarii. White pepper was priced at seven denarii and black pepper at four denarii per pound. He complains that, because of the import of pepper, the drain on the Roman Empire was 50 million sesterces[24] per annum. He laments thus in Natural History:

> It is quite surprising that the use of pepper has come so much into fashion, seeing that in other substances which we use, it is sometimes their sweetness, and sometimes their appearance that has attracted our notice; whereas, pepper has nothing in it that can plead as a recommendation to either fruit or berry, its only desirable quality being a certain pungency; and yet it is for this that we import it all the way from India! Who was the first to make trial of it as an article of food? and who, I wonder, was the man that was not content to prepare himself by hunger only for the satisfying of a greedy appetite?

(N.H. 12.14)

The conquest of Egypt by the Romans c. 30 BC opened the sea route from the Indian Malabar coast to Alexandria on the Red Sea. Strabo, the ancient Roman geographer, makes mention of a fleet of around 120 ships making an annual trip to India and back using the newly discovered monsoon current.

---

24   Sesterces was a Roman coin. The value of this coin changed with the economic condition prevailing during the time. One sesterces value in today's terms is estimated to have varied from half a US dollar to six dollars.

Pepper was an ingredient in the spicy wine popular in ancient Rome. Black pepper had widespread use as a food seasoning across the Roman Empire. Apicius' De re coquinaria, a 3rd century AD cookbook, has pepper as an ingredient in most recipes popular during that period. It was a favorite in the cuisine of the rich and famous.

Pepper was so valuable that it was accepted as collateral or even currency. Alaric the Visigoth and Attila the Hun each demanded from Rome a ransom of more than a ton of pepper when they besieged the city in 5th century AD.

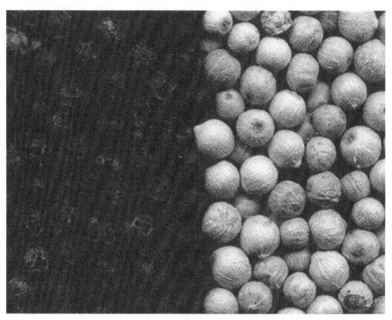

Picture 17 Black and white dried peppercorns
Photo by Bunchofgrapes

Before the days of refrigeration and the invention of other food preservatives, pepper and salt were extensively used to both flavor and preserve food until milder spices and herbs slowly replaced black pepper only in the 17th century. This culinary innovation was introduced first in French cuisine.

Trade and Commerce

With the decline of the Roman Empire, the lucrative trade in spices that included pepper moved from the hands of the Arab traders to Europeans. Venice and Constantinople became the hub for onward export into Europe. The Dutch were the first spice traders followed by the Portuguese. The colonization of India by the British led to a spice trade monopoly falling in their hands.

Huge amounts of pepper were consumed by ancient Roman and European societies. Recipes for pepper sauces can be seen in Roman
novels of the 1stcentury AD. This was one of the most sought-after spice of the time. Its popularity endured right through to the Middle Ages.

Advancement in navigation methods, improved safety of maritime vessels and resulted in reduction of logistic risk. This led to a reduction in the price of spices and other products. The monopoly of India as the natural commodity producer of spices broke as alternate production areas in Southeast Asia were discovered and gained importance. Increased supply led to further decline in prices. Low spice cuisine changes in European food led to further reduction in demand.

Discovery of alternate food preservatives further reduced demand of spices and herbs as preservative. Still, despite the drop in the price of spices, pepper continues to be an important spice. It is still preferred in cuisine across the globe. Pepper is now grown and traded across a wide and diversified production region. This includes India, Malaysia, Indonesia, China, Vietnam, Brazil, and Sri Lanka.

In 2013, the global pepper production was put at 472,526 metric tons. Vietnam is now the biggest producer having produced 163,000 metric tons of pepper in 2013, followed by Indonesia with 88,700 metric tons and India with 53,000 metric tons (all figures are FAO statistic estimates).

Essential Oil

Black pepper yields a warm and spicy essential oil with a smell that is faintly reminiscent of clove oil, albeit, a bit more refined. It is light amber to yellow-green in color with watery viscosity. Unripe, sundried peppercorns are subjected to steam distillation to produce the essential oil.
The yield is approximately 2%.

The essential oil is composed of the following chemical constituents: a-thujone, a-pinene, camphene, sabinene, b-pinene, a-phellandrene, myrcene, limonene, caryophyllene, b-farnesene, b-bisabolene, linalool, and terpinen-4-ol. The oil contains, in addition to alkaloids, moisture, protein, minerals, fiber, and carbohydrates. It is rich in vitamin B-complex and contains traces of calcium, iron, and phosphorus.

Black pepper oil may cause irritation to sensitive skin. Its excessive use can over stimulate the kidneys. The oil helps increase warmth
of the body and mind. It relieves sore muscles and joints, boosts the immune and digestive systems, stimulates the kidneys, and disperses bruising by increasing circulation in affected areas of the skin. Black pepper has a pungent, crisp aroma that is said to be comforting and energizing.

Black pepper oil can be used for pain relief, rheumatism, chills, flu, colds, increasing circulation, reducing exhaustion, muscular aches, physical and emotional coldness, nerve tonic, and fevers.

The oil has a strong, sharp, spicy aroma which adds an "intriguing" note when blended into aromatherapy bath and body care products. It is often used with thyme to create cosmetic products like body lotions, creams, etc. Black pepper oil blends well with frankincense, sandalwood, lavender, rosemary, marjoram, and other citrus and floral oils.

In Healing

In addition to its use in cuisine, pepper is regarded for its medicinal properties too. In India, a decoction of black pepper powder, ginger, and sugar is a common home remedy for cough and cold. Tea infused with black pepper and ginger helps reduce discomfort from the common cold.

Ayurvedic medicine with black pepper as an ingredient is said to treat a range of diseases like cholera, toothache, dysentery, and conditions of the respiratory and digestive systems. Pepper increases the flow of saliva, stimulates appetite, encourages peristalsis, and tones the colon muscles. These are properties typical to most spices.

In Ayurveda, black pepper is a healing spice. It is often used along with long pepper and ginger, a combination said to have cleansing and antioxidant properties. Pepper is a bioavailability enhancer.

Pepper enhances the flow of oxygen to the brain, improves digestion and circulation, and stimulates the appetite. It excites the salivary and the sweat glands, besides killing intestinal worms. It helps propel downward movement of the abdominal wind.

Black pepper is also one of the few spices which Ayurveda describes as pramathi (helping to open obstruction in different channels of the body). Black pepper, as mentioned earlier, is added to turmeric and many other herbal formulations as an activator.

Scientists have made efforts to validate the traditional herbal remedies used in Ayurveda, Siddha, and Unani systems. Experiments conducted by Karsha et al. (2010) shows the antibacterial action of pepper on a variety of bacteria ranging from Staphyloccocus sps, Pseudomonas, etc.

Study conducted on mice shows spasmodic (cholinergic) and anti-spasmodic effects, action like loperamide and nifedipine. Pepper and piperine can be used to treat gastrointestinal motility disorders (Mehmood et al., 2010).

The biological role of Piper nigrum has been studied and its action observed by Ahmed et al. in 2012. They found that Piper nigrum has many properties: anti-apoptotic, antibacterial, anti-colon toxin, anti-depressant, anti-fungal, anti-diarrheal, anti-inflammatory, anti-mutagenic, anti-metastatic activity, antioxidative, anti-pyretic, anti-spasmodic, anti-tumor, anti-thyroid, ciprofloxacin potentiator, cold extremities, hepatoprotective, etc.

It is widely used in various herbal cough syrups. It is also used in anti-inflammatory, anti-malarial, anti-leukemia treatment (Nahak et al., 2011). Black pepper is said to help bring about improvements in the conditions of poor concentration and ameliorates an apprehensive state of mind.

MALABATHRUM, OR INDIAN BAY LEAF (Cinnamomum tamala) leaves that spice your food

It is an Indian spice used mainly in South Asia. To the ancient Romans and Greeks, it was known as malabathrum or the malabar leaf. Malabar is a region is located on the West Coast of South India. However, malabathrum is not found in the Malabar, a contradiction that will be explained later in this chapter. In India, the North Indian name of the spice is tej patta. The botanical name of the species is Cinnamomum tamala (alternatively called as Cinnamomum tejpata).

This is a small tree that grows rarely over eight meters in height. The Sanskrit name for the tree is tamālapattram, literally translated as "dark- tree leaves." The Greeks adopted a modification of the Sanskrit name and called it malabathrum or malobathrum.

The plant grows in the Himalayan foothills in North East India. The Indian bay leaf is twice as long as the bay laurel leaf and has an olive-green color.

There are three prominent veins running down the length of the leaf compared to just one in the bay laurel leaf. The foliage of the Indian bay leaf looks quite like that of cinnamon.

Due to the relatively restricted geographical distribution of tej patta and its extensive use in cuisine of North and East India, Bangladesh, and Nepal, the species has been overexploited leading to substantial diminishing of the number of plants. As it is a slow-growing species, the economics of raising the species as an agro-forestry crop is not attractive enough. Meanwhile, its population continues to diminish in its habitat.

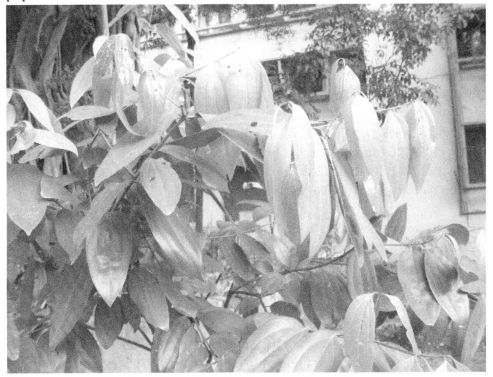

Picture 18 Cinnamomum tamala
Photo: Sudhir Ahluwalia

C. tamala does not find favor as a plantation species in forest plantations.

But, in Nepal, the species is planted and exploited as an important non-timber forest product. Choudhury et al. (2014) has noted that large scale plantations of tej patta have been raised in Udayapur district of Nepal. Lower wage cost and few livelihood alternatives have made it possible for this species to emerge as a viable non-timber forest product crop in that country. The ready market of India has made it possible for growers and traders to earn a small income from these plantations.

Trade and Commerce

Periplus Maris Erytraei[25] mentions malabathrum leaves as one of the major exports to Ancient Rome. The trade took place from the Tamil kingdoms of South India. The leaves were said to have been sourced from people with mongoloid features that they called Sesatai, who brought the produce to the town market from where it was purchased by traders.

In ancient times, people residing in villages adjoining the forests in Northeast India collected these leaves and brought them to the village markets for sale, a practice that continues to this day. The banks of the Ganges River in the region had many such village markets.

River transportation was, at that time, the preferred mode of transport as it was less hazardous than land routes. Boats with tej patta leaves took the river route to the Hooghly Port. From there, the merchandise would move to other ports on India's eastern coast for onward journey to Greece, Rome, and Egypt.

An active and close interaction between the Indians and the Greeks existed from 4th century BC to 1st century AD. Commerce was quite well organized during the period. Traders' guilds effectively managed business and commerce, and the state collected its share of taxes, letting trade go unhindered.

---

25   The Periplus Maris Erythraei (or "Voyage around the Erythraean Sea") is an anonymous work from around the middle of the 1st century CE. It is said to have been written by a Greek-speaking Egyptian merchant.

Arthasastra, the political treatise written by Kautilya, and the stone edicts of Emperor Ashoka give us a good insight into governing and trade practices that existed during this period.

Sea routes connected West Indian ports to Egypt too. The list of India's exports to Egypt comprised ivory, tortoise-shell, pearls, unguents, and dyes (especially indigo), nard, costus, malabathrum, long pepper, iron, and wood, especially teak.

Spices were in high demand, first by the Greeks and Egyptians, and then the Romans. These were used as perfume, incense, condiment, and medicine. The South Indian ports on the West Coast from Gujarat to Cape Comorin extensively participated in this trade to the West. There are references to export of malabathrum to Roman dominions from Indian Southern ports of Muziris, which I find quite unconvincing.

We know that cinnamon, cassia, camphor, green cardamom, pepper, etc. were exported to the Mediterranean from the southern ports on the West Coast. For the Indian bay leaf produce from East India to come to these ports, the leaves would have had to circumvent the entire peninsular coast to reach the West Coast, the logistics alone making the cost of this spice prohibitive.

It is more likely that locally growing cinnamon leaves were sold as malabathrum and shipped to Rome and the Mediterranean region. Having lived in both South and North India, I can vouch that even in this day, we would rather use cinnamon leaves in our cuisine than try and discover true malabrathum brought over a thousand miles away from Eastern Himalayan region.

Trade in Indian bay leaves appears to have continued unabated up to the middle of the 1st millennium AD. Some medieval recipes for beer brewing mention folia which could be malabathrum. The land route to Persia and onward to Greece got disrupted with the demise of the Roman Empire. Trade connection to the west from the northern regions of India would have suffered due to the political uncertainty in the region.

Northeastern India, home to the malabathrum, was rediscovered only in the Age of Exploration, when Western scholars, for the first time, arrived in India and studied its products. In the 16th century, Garcia de Orta encountered the leaves while traveling in India and identified them as the malabathrum spice from ancient records.

In Food

In ancient Greece and Rome, the leaves were used to prepare fragrant oil, called Oleum Malabathri. The Romans used them in both perfumery and food. Roman cookery books called them folia (leaves), a reference often confused with the Mediterranean bay leaves. The Greeks used the leaves to flavor wine along with absinth wormwood. The Roman food specialist Gaius Gavius Apicus mentions malabathrum as one of the good kitchen spices.

Trade of the Indian bay leaf resumed in the Middle Ages. Disruption of trade due to war made the ancient trade routes passing through Asia into Europe unsafe. This led to cessation in trade between India and Europe. The name probably continued to be used in mediaeval texts to describe the dried leaves of several trees from the genus Cinnamomum that produces cinnamon. The leaves of these trees are also aromatic and continue to be used in food and medicine.

Malabathrum leaves were used in unguents. Unguents were ointments made from medicinal herbs ground into the form of a paste, mixed with water and oil. These were applied to affected parts of the body like sores, cuts, wounds, and inflammations. Unguents were popular with ancient healers across the globe. Malabathrum leaves give an aroma like cinnamon and can often be confused with each other. Cinnamon leaves are also used as spice in South Asian cuisine. The Indian bay leaf was a favorite of the Mughals and continue to be extensively and almost exclusively used in the kitchens of Northern India. In Mughal cuisine, tej patta (malabathrum or Indian bay leaf) is used along with cinnamon, cloves, and cardamom in the rice dish called biryani.

122

Indian bay leaves are very popular in the Terai plains of Southern Nepal too. Food in the Terai is less spicy when compared to North Indian cuisine. Indian bay leaves are a key flavor to the many vegetarian curries of that area, particularly the Mithila region around Janakpur. The Indian bay leaves are used in Northeast India, bordering Burma. There, these are often sold fresh perhaps in a manner that is no different from that observed in the 1st century AD and described in the Greek text Periplus Maris Erytraei.

In Medicine

Indian bay leaf has a very cinnamon-like aroma which is different from the Mediterranean bay laurel leaf. The aroma of the bay laurel leaf resembles pine and lemon. Essential oil extracted from the Indian bay leaves contains monoterpenoids including phellandrene, eugenol, linalool, and some traces of alpha-pinene, pcymene, beta-pinene, limonene, and phenyl propanoids (Ahmed et al., 2000).

The main medicinal action of the plant is its ability to reduce blood sugar, validated by experiments on rats and comparable to that of the anti-diabetic modern drug Glibenclamide (Chakraborty et al., 2010). These studies raise the likelihood of its probable use as an adjunct medicine for treating diabetes (Kumar et al., 2012).

The plant is also known to reduce cholesterol levels in rats (Dhulasawant et al., 2010; and AL-Mamun et al., 2011). It has nephro-protective properties (Ullah et al., 2013). Other medicinal properties of the plant include anti-diarrheal, hepato-protective, gastro-protective, antibacterial, immunomodulatory, insecticidal, etc. (Thamizhselvam et al., 2012).

Trials to test the analgesic property of the plant have indicated that its affect could be better than modern drugs like indomethacin and aspirin. B caryophyllene, linalool, caryophyllene oxide, and other alkaloids have been isolated from the plant. The leaves are rich in antioxidants.

Tej patta in Ayurveda is used to correct ailments of the digestive system. It is regarded as an herbal remedy for piles. It helps alleviate nausea and vomiting. It is said to increase appetite and is a remedy in cold, cough, and coryza.

CARDAMOM- the antioxidant spice

There are two varieties of cardamom. Large or big cardamom and a small pod variety—green cardamom. Big cardamom is also called black cardamom, Bengal cardamom, or Siamese cardamom and belongs to the Amomum genus. The smaller variety is from Elettaria genus. Both Amomum and Elettaria genus belong to the same Zingiberaceae family. Ginger is another popular spice that belongs to this family.

Besides India, cardamom is grown as a commercial crop in Guatemala. On a smaller scale, cardamom is also cultivated in Tanzania, Sri Lanka, El Salvador, Vietnam, Laos, Thailand, Cambodia, Honduras, and Papua & New Guinea.

Black cardamom pods are dark and smoky with high tones of camphor and mint. There are two species of Amomum that yield the large cardamom fruit. These species are Amomum aromaticum and Amomum subulatum.

This is an evergreen monocot shrub with large ovate spathe-like leaves. Shrub height is around five feet. Its fruit is borne in spikes. Spikes emerge directly from the rhizome. The species is cultivated under shade of trees in natural tropical evergreen ecosystems. These form the under storey of the forest. Amomum aromaticum or Bengal cardamom fruits are often adulterated with a cheaper variety from Amomum subulatum plants.

The other major cardamom species is the true cardamom or green cardamom. This has a distinct minty aroma. Green cardamom is cultivated in South India's Western Ghats region. It is also grown in Malaysia.

Green cardamom is cultivated under the shade of large evergreen trees. Evergreen forests are multi-storeyed forests. Cardamom plantations are raised in the under storey. The plants love shade and thrive in filtered light that can penetrate through the thick canopy formed by large trees.

Cardamom cultivation does not cause any major destruction of the delicate evergreen forest ecosystem. To cultivate a cardamom crop, no removal of the upper storey trees is required. The multi-storeyed ecosystem can continue to grow largely undisturbed. Green cardamom plants rarely attain a height beyond two to three meters.

Cardamom pods after harvesting are dried in the sun. These are bleached with sulfur fumes to give the pod a pleasing green color.

Historical References

Cardamom was used by ancient Sumerians as revealed by the Cuneiform tablets discovered from the Library of Ashurbanipal (688-633 BC). It was a prized plant. There is mention of it being raised in the garden of Merodach Baladan (721-702 BC).

Cardamom was imported into Sumeria from India. Archeological evidence to the existence of this trade goes back to the Indus Valley Civilization period (2800-1800 BC). Recent excavations in India indicate that the civilization existed as far back as 4000 BC. There are references to the use of cardamom in the sacrificial fires of the Vedic people in the Krishna Yajurveda text Taitreya samhita.

Cardamom is mentioned as a medicinal plant in Charakasamhita. These compilations are said to consolidate medicinal practices that go as far back to the 8th century BC.

Kautilya mentions the use of cardamom in his political work, Arthashastra (4thcentury BC). Cardamom use is mentioned by Theophrastus (c. 310 BC) too. He says of cardamom and amomom, "Some say they come from Iran, others from India, like spikenard and so many other aromatics" (Historia

Plantarum). These, along with other plant aromatics, were extensively used by the Greeks and Romans in perfume and medicine.

Ancient Egyptians burnt the dried seeds for incense. It was also used in combination with resinous substances, herbs, and spices. The incense was used in their ancient temples and palaces. Cardamom was one of the most important spices imported into the Mediterranean region. There are references to the existence of such a trade in the Bible.

The destruction of the Jewish temple in Jerusalem and the trade in spices are beautifully and poignantly captured in the Book of Revelation in the Bible. An extract is as follows:

Revelation 18:13

"Cinnamon, cardamom, incense, myrrh, frankincense, wine, oil, flour, grain, cattle, sheep, horses, chariots—and bodies—and people's souls."

In Medicine

Metopion is the name of an Egyptian ointment popular with the Ancient Egyptians and Greeks. Diosocrides mentions that Metopion is the name of an Egyptian plant from which galbanum was derived. The ointment consists of the oil of bitter almonds and unripe olives scented with cardamom, sweet rush, sweet flag, honey, wine, myrrh, seed of balsamum, galbanum, and turpentine resin. According to Dioscorides, the best Metopion was the one that smelt more of cardamom and myrrh than of galbanum.

In medicine the ointment was to be heat- and sweat-producing, and was used to "open the vessels," draw and purge ulcers, and to treat cut sinews and muscles. Spices, in general, are stimulating to the senses, help in digestion, and enhance sense of well-being.

Cardamom was used as a tooth cleaner by the Ancient Egyptians. It was used in perfume by the Greeks and Romans. The ancient Greeks, around the

4thcentury BC and subsequently, the Romans, highly valued cardamom as a culinary spice.

It was a base for herbal medicines. It was regarded as a digestive aid, a property that is also recognized in Ayurveda. It is common in India today to brew tea with cardamom, ginger, and other spices during winter to keep the body warm and comfortable.

Spices were symbols of royalty and luxury. Cardamom was one of the ingredients of the legendary all-cure potion mithridatium or theriake, said to have been concocted by Mithradates VI, sovereign of Pontus (120-63 BC).

Mithridates VI is said to have ruled the region of Armenia and Turkey. The potion is said to contain 54-60 ingredients that included cardamom. This remedy, detailed by many ancient herbal medicine works such as Aulus Cornelius Celsus's De Medicina, was claimed to cure a person of an assortment of ills. It was also taken as a universal antidote to any and all poisons. Research in modern times has discredited most of these ancient potions.

Small cardamom (Elleteria sps) was observed to reduce blood pressure in stage 1 hypertensive individuals. It also helps reduce the tendency of blood clot formation and raise the antioxidant levels in the body (Verma et all, 2009). Cardamom extract was seen to inhibit human platelet aggregation (Suneetha et al., 2005). Verma et al., (2010) found Amomum subulatum to be a cardio-adaptogen against physical stress.

It is a diuretic with sedative action (Gilani et al., 2008). They believe that the ability to lower blood pressure is due to diuretic and sedative property of the species. The antioxidant effect of the bark and black cardamom seed was also observed in an experiment conducted on rats fed on a high-fat diet (Dhuley, 1999) . The antioxidant property of cardamom was observed to vary with variety (Amma et al., 2010).

The anti-convulsant and sedative property of an Ayurvedic formulation

Unmadnashak Ghrita which has Elletaria cardamomum, Gardenia gummifera, Ferula narthex, Bacopa monneri, and cow's clarified butter was observed in an experiment conducted on mice (Achliya et al., 2004).

The anti-microbial action of cardamom oil against one or more bacterial species was observed in studies (Kubo et al., 1991; Supriya et al., 2012; and Kumar et al., 2010). The antibacterial action of the dry cardamom fruit extract was observed in various other studies also (Kaushik et al., 2010; Jazila et al., 2007; and Hussain et al., 2011). The anti-microbial activity of both large and small cardamom plants was observed against microorganisms causing dental caries (Aneja et al., 2011). Cold extracts of Amomum subulatum were observed to be effective against Pseudomonas aeruginosa, a hospital-infection causing organism (Jain et al., 1976).

The plant is said to provide relief in cases of stomach disorders, improved appetite, and digestion. The fruit and seed were seen to be anti-spasmodic and analgesic. The action of cardamom oil was found to be anti-spasmodic (Al- Zuhair et al., 1996). The analgesic property of Amomum subulatum was observed by Shukla et al. (2010), and its anti-inflammatory activity was evaluated by Alam et al. (2011).

Herbal healers claim that the spice helps cure malaria, pulmonary tuberculosis, is a curative for throat inflammation, congestion of lungs, that it reduces inflammation of eyelids, and is a general mouth freshener.

Experiments on rabbits validate the anti-asthmatic property of the species (Khan et al., 2011). In Unani medicine, cardamom is used to treat gastric ulcers and other gastric ailments. A study conducted on rats showed a gastroprotective effect of cardamom (Elettaria cardamomum). The size of gastric lesions was observed to reduce and the actions were observed to be similar to ranitidine. The anti-ulcerogenic activity of Elettaria cardamomum and Ammomum subulatum was studied and the property validated (Jafri et al., 2001; and Farah et al., 2005). The methanolic extracts of A. subulatum seeds were seen to possess a hepatoprotective property (Parmar et al., 2009).

Essential oil from small cardamom (Elletaria cardamomum) seeds was shown to possess an anti-feedant property against insects indicating that it could be developed as an insecticide (Huang et al., 2000). The large cardamom (Amomum subulatum) fruits were observed to possess properties that help reduce sugar levels in the blood of experimental rats (Vavaiya et al., 2010).

The fruit is rich in essential oils and flavonoids. They are also used as a mouth wash, cure toothache, gingivitis, and parodontosis.

Cardamom in Chinese Medicine

In traditional Chinese medicine, the Amomum varieties are usually employed in much the same manner as the Elettaria variants. The Chinese liberally employ black cardamom in the creation of alcoholic or alcohol-based tonics and potions. Black cardamom is typically ground into a paste and mixed with honey or some other sweet syrup for relief from bronchitis or asthma.

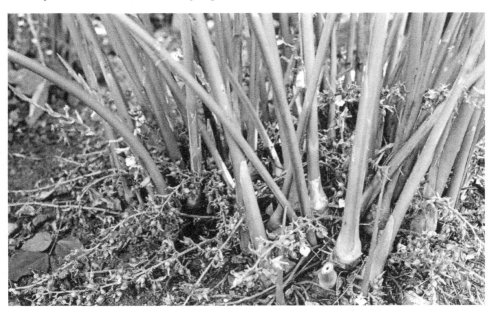

Picture 19 Elettaria cardamomum plants
Photo: Dr Ravikumar, Senior Botanist, FRLHT

This same syrup may also be employed as a temporary disinfectant for wounds, or as an anti-gangrene and antibacterial remedy for open wounds and injuries both prior to and after suturing or cauterization. Very strong decoctions of black cardamom are employed to disinfect bandages.

Black cardamom mixed with tea (usually the "red" (black) or oolong varieties) is typically drunk after meals. They are said to help with digestion and aid in nutrient absorption. Cardamom is added to milk tea in India. Other exotic practices in China include drinking of black tea with cardamom, at times mixed with lu rong (prepared deer antler, usually of the Cervus sika species), don sen(Campanumea pilosula), and orange or mandarin peel. It is typically given as remedy for anemia, general weakness, wasting diseases (i.e., tuberculosis), and malaria.

Tinctures made of pure cardamom are rare. Alcoholic beverages with cardamom or its use as an aromatic and flavoring additive are common in traditional Chinese medicine. These "flavored liquors" are said to help boost immunity, improve digestion, purify and tonify the blood, and increase vigor. Practices like traditional Chinese medicine are also observed in Ayurveda.

Cardamom in Ayurveda

Cardamom is widely used for relief in digestion-related ailments. In India, green cardamom is used to treat infections in the teeth and gums. The spice is also used to prevent and treat throat troubles, get relief from congestion of the lungs and pulmonary tuberculosis as well as to reduce inflammation of eyelids. It is also reportedly used as an antidote against both snake and scorpion venom.

Due to its ability to improve assimilation of nutrients and to hasten the metabolic rate, cardamom has now been incorporated into some diet and weight-loss beverages. Being a remedy for anemia, it is believed to also be an excellent nutrition supplement.

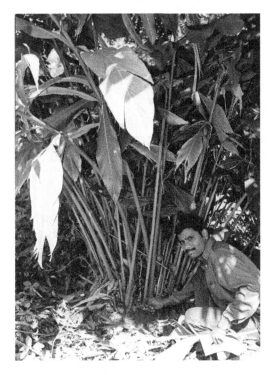

Picture 20 Amomum subulatum
Photo: Dr Ravikumar, Senior Botanist, FRLHT

Cardamom Essential Oil

The whole or ground seeds, when allowed to steep in oil, are used to treat topical dermatitis, allergies, and fungal infections. When combined with warming spices or herbs that improve circulation, the macerated oil may be employed for massage as a relief from the pains and aches of arthritis or rheumatism. It is also said to boost hair growth and scalp health by improving circulation and curing topical fungal-based ailments such as dandruff. The essential oil possesses the same properties as the seed, albeit, in a more concentrated state.

The essential oil is used for its uplifting and invigorating properties. It aids digestion, removes flatulence, and treats nausea. It is also regarded as an aphrodisiac. It helps counter irritation during premenstrual tension. It is useful in alleviating symptoms of cough, cold, and sore throat.

In Food

With the fall of the Roman Empire, the center of trade moved away from Asia to Europe. Venice and Istanbul, the latter then called Constantinople, became the new centers through which flowed pepper, cloves, cinnamon, etc. This continued through the Middle Ages.

The Vikings came across cardamom about 1,000 years ago in Constantinople and introduced it to Scandinavia, where it remains popular to this day. In the Scandinavian countries, it is used in baked goods and confectionaries. In Europe and North America, it is an ingredient in curry powder and in some sausage products. The Portuguese, the Dutch, and finally the British, took control of the trade between Asia and Europe (16th to 19th century AD). Valerius first distilled the essential oil in 1544.

Despite its numerous applications in the cuisine of Sri Lanka, India, and Iran, 60% of the world production is exported to the Arab (Southwest Asia, North Africa) countries, where it is widely used to flavor coffee. Cardamom infused coffee is served in tiny cups and slowly sipped. Bedouins (Arabic nomads) are known to keep capsules of cardamom in the spouts of coffee pots. Each time the coffee is poured, it gets flavored by the spice.

Cardamom-scented coffee is popular in Ethiopia too. Coffee beans are roasted just before usage, often mixed with spices like cloves, cardamom, etc. Once the roast mix is cool, it is ground and brewed. Other flavors like fresh leaves of rue are also added. It is mentioned as an aphrodisiac in the Arabian nights.

Cardamom is best stored in the pod form because once the seeds are exposed or ground, they quickly lose their flavor. In India, the large pod cardamom is used in biryani. Cardamom is also used as an ingredient in curry masala. Black cardamom is exclusively employed to season food, especially meat-based dishes. It is also used in medicated potions, elixirs, and tonics.

Green cardamom is used to flavor desserts and as a mouth freshener after meals. It is said to detoxify caffeine in coffee. Its wide applications lead to it being called the Queen of Spices.

Cardamom oil is used to flavor processed foods, liqueurs, perfumery, and confectionary. The essential oil is often used in combination with the oils of orange, cinnamon, cloves, and caraway to provide a distinctive flavor to baked goods, coffee, etc.
In Chinese cuisine, black cardamom is used extensively for flavor and seasoning, in combination with other herbs and spices. Black cardamom also features in several regional liquor recipes.

Cardamom is used to flavor alcoholic beverages. Finely ground cardamom seeds are mixed with tobacco or marijuana for flavor. It is mixed with spices like cloves, holy basil and used as substitute for mentholated tobacco. The spice tobacco mixture is used in pipes or hookahs.

In Cosmetics

Cardamom oil is extracted from seed by the steam distillation process. The volatile oil contains borneol, camphor, pinene, selinene, limonene, eugenol, and a range of other alkaloids. The aroma of cardamom essential oil is warm-spicy, sweet, somewhat floral, and camphorates.

It is used as a bath oil, food flavor, and in burners and vaporizers. Cardamom oil is a popular after spray due to its refined, spicy, and edgy notes. This oil is a mild stimulant with a sensual quality and makes a light, refreshing bath oil.

The oil is clear, pale yellow in color and relatively expensive. The aroma can be intoxicating, and when combined with Yang yang, cardamom makes a highly beneficial oil to alleviate depression.

The seeds are chewed to sweeten the breath. Cleopatra is said to have burnt cardamom incense whenever Mark Anthony visited her. The essential oil of cardamom was a central ingredient in many ancient perfumes. It was quite popular in Ancient Egypt and Rome for its warm, slightly floral aroma for which reasons it was used as a natural aphrodisiac.

According to herbs.com, in magic, hoodoo, and voodoo practices, cardamom seeds are typically carried in juju bags alongside other "love-inviting" herbs or spices to help attract potential lovers or to incite lust and desire. Ground seeds were incorporated into both alcoholic and non-alcoholic beverages with the aim to incite desire, increase libido, or elicit lust.

Within the collective body of shamanic practices and some schools of ceremonial magic, cardamom seeds are employed more for purifications and protection—either burnt as incense or housed in medicine pouches— as the physical properties of the spice is claimed to have the ability to rejuvenate and cleanse the body.

Production and Trade

Cardamom was one of the spices that was subjected to import tax in Alexandria in 126 AD. Alexandria, with the Romans occupying most of North Africa and the Mediterranean region and beyond, had become a major port at which much of the trade in the entire region was conducted. Cardamom, like other major spices coming from India, was considered a luxury and an import tax was levied.

According to the figures of the Multicommodity Exchange of India, Guatemala is the largest cardamom producing country today followed by India producing between 30,000 to 38,000 metric tons per annum.[26] Guatemala produces green cardamom and exports most of it. In 2012-13, as per provisional trade estimates, India's production was estimated to be around 12,000 MT (Spices Board of India).

---

26   www.guatemalacardamom.com

Consumption of cardamom has increased sharply throughout the world during the last two decades. The major consumers are the Middle Eastern countries, India, Pakistan, Europe, the US, and Japan. The Middle East accounts for more than 60% of the world's consumption

CHAPTER V

HERBS IN CHINESE CUISINE

Herbs and spices are an integral part of traditional Chinese cooking and medicine. Huang di Neijing (The Yellow Emperor's Classic on Medicine) is said to be more than 2,000 years old, dated to the Han Dynasty era (206 BC-220 AD). This tome is about acupuncture, and human health and medicine. Huang di Neijing takes a holistic look at human life, and the emphasis is on achieving a balance of the life forces, qi, yin, and yang[27] and the body fluids. The work is in the form of questions and answers between the Yellow Emperor Huang di and his acupuncturist Qi Bo.

Food is integral to healing in Chinese medicine. Traditional Chinese medicine links well-being to consuming food appropriate to the season and health of the individual. In summer, yin foods like melon and cucumber should be eaten as they help cool the body. In winter, yang foods like garlic and onions are recommended. These stimulate the system and help keep energy levels high.

Eating the appropriate food helps to maintain nutritional well-being. It also helps heal a sick body. Herbs appropriate to the winter like garlic and onions help combat cold and flu. Yang herbs like ginger and garlic also help in the digestion process.

Summer foods like melons, cucumber, and cooling drinks made from unripe mango (recommended in Ayurveda) help prevent sunstroke and keep the body cool. In Imperial China, wealthy households had herbalists who made recommendations on the appropriate foods and herbs during a season.

---

27   Yin and Yang are two opposites like sky and earth, day and night, active and passive. Literally speaking, yin represents the dark side of a slope and yang, the sunny side. While yang brings energy, brightness, and activity to a person, yin does the oppositive. Disbalance of these leads to disease and sickness.

There are five basic flavors mentioned in Chinese cuisine: acrid or pungent, sweet, bitter, sour, and salty. It is the balance of these flavors that defines the cuisine of the many regions of China. In Chinese cuisine, the focus on spices is lesser than in Indian food.

The most popular herb-and-spice combination in Chinese cuisine is the Five Spice Powder, a combination of cassia, star anise, cloves, fennel, and Sichuan peppercorns.

Ginger, onion, anise seed, black cardamom, licorice root, nutmeg, rice powder, cilantro, mustard, orange peel, and black pepper are some of the other herbs and spices used in Chinese cuisine. Chili was introduced to the world from Latin America and grew in popularity across the world. It has now become an important ingredient in many Chinese sauces. Chili is often used in combination with Szechwan peppers.

In Chinese tradition, there is no clearly defined line distinguishing food from medicine. Traditional Chinese kitchens frequently use medicinal herbs like ginseng, astragalus, wolfberry, and jujube in addition to the spices in food to prevent disease and degeneration.

Herb combinations called constitutional herbs are used to balance forces of yin and yang in the body. Balance keeps the body healthy. Other herbs, called tonic herbs, help boost immunity and increase resistance.

GARLIC and its myriad medicinal properties

Garlic in Chinese is called "suan." It, along with ginger, is one of the two integral spices of Chinese cooking. Sheng Nung's (c. 2700 BC) treatise is the earliest documented evidence on the use of garlic in China.

There is a lot of debate on the origin of garlic. Some scholars claim that it came to Asia from Sumeria with traders (c. 2600-2100 BC). According to kew.org the plant origins lie in Central Asia. I think, like many other plant species, garlic's original geographic distribution was not restricted to one or two locations.

Allium sativum is the cultivated species of garlic. Some scholars claim that the species may have descended from Allium longicuspis. This species is observed growing in the wild in the Central Asian and neighboring Southwest Asian region. There are, though, many other wild garlic species found in other parts of the world.

Allium vineale found in North America is the wild garlic used by North American Indians. Allium canadense is another wild garlic species found growing in fields of North America. Allium ursinum is wild garlic found in the UK.

It is observed across a wide geographic range from Central Asia, northern parts of South Asia across to the Sumerian region (modern day Iraq). There are multiple references to garlic in the Bible, Ancient Egyptian, and Greek writings supporting the wide geographic distribution theory.

Garlic was locally produced and consumed. Unlike for pepper, cinnamon, and other spices that were imported into the Mediterranean region, I did not come across any ancient references to the import of garlic to any of major centers of ancient civilizations of Asia and the Mediterranean region.

Garlic belongs to the Alliaceae family. There are said to be around 300 varieties of garlic. A garlic bulb is composed of several bulbils. In trade, these are called cloves. A single garlic bulb could have up to 20 bulbils.

The plant grows to a height of 2 feet. A flowering shoot called the scape grows from the base and flowers are arranged on top of the scape forming a globose head. Scapes are pinched off early to prevent diversion of nutrition away from the bulb.

The plant has been in use as a spice for over 3,000 years in China, Egypt, Greece, Rome, and India. Garlic was found in the palace at Knossos (dated between 1400 and 1800 BC) in Crete, and the Egyptian pyramids where well-preserved garlic cloves were recovered from the tomb of King Tutankhamen.

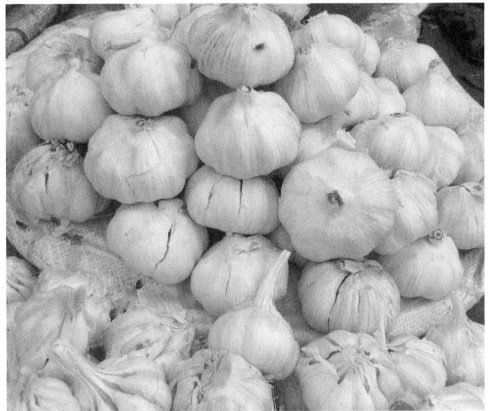

Picture 21: Garlic
Photo: Sudhir Ahluwalia

Garlic's initial use was probably as a food preservative. The strong flavor of garlic would have helped mask foul odor emanating from food stored for extended periods. To fresh food, it added flavor and taste. Garlic, over time, has become part of daily human diet across the globe.

Food

Garlic is an essential ingredient of Chinese food. Garlic preserve is used as an accompaniment to dumplings. Garlic is an important spice in Szechuan food and is a yang food. In Northeast China, garlic is preserved in rice vinegar, sugar and salt. This is ritually done on the 8th of December, a date that denotes the formal commencement of winter.

Garlic is popular in Indian cuisine too, commonly used to season lentil and other curries. Garlic is valued for its digestive properties and is sold in capsule form as an over-the-counter nutraceutical product. Garlic capsules are popular with people suffering from flatulence and gastric disorders.

Leaves and flowers have a milder flavor when compared to the bulb and are eaten when the plant is young and the shoot still tender. The only inedible part is the papery skin covering the cloves.

Leaves and the scape are often used in curries or stir-fried food. Cloves are also eaten after roasting. Garlic, mixed with oil or butter, is used to flavor bread. Garlic toast, garlic bread, canapés, etc. are some popular snacks. Garlic bulbs, when fermented at high temperature, turn black with a sweet and syrupy taste, and is a preferred condiment in Korean food.

Mixed with sugar, salt, and other spices or vegetables like onion and tomato, garlic is a popular seasoning spice. The shoots can be pickled and eaten as an appetizer. The taste of garlic powder is different from fresh garlic, but it can be used as a substitute to fresh garlic. Garlic oil is produced by frying garlic cloves in oil, and the aromatic oil, upon cooling, is used in cuisine. Garlic-flavored sauces are quite popular across the globe.

In Ancient Egypt, Ancient Greece, and Rome, garlic was fed to workers as it enhances strength and stamina. Soldiers too would eat garlic before battle.

There are references to Jewish slaves being fed garlic and onions in the Bible. It was a popular spice in the region with the Jews being particularly fond of garlic. Tradition has it that when the Jews led by Moses fled Egypt crossing the Red Sea in search of the Holy Land, in the desert they missed vegetables, spices, and other food that they ate in Egypt. This is evident from the following verse, Numbers 11:5 (NKJV), which states the Jews missed "the fish, the cucumbers and the melons and the leeks, and the onions and the garlic."

Due to its pungent odor, garlic was avoided as food by the rich in ancient India. Buddhists and Jains did not eat garlic. Some of them refrain from eating garlic even today. As Buddhist influence spread across Asia, garlic lost some of its popular appeal in this region. Even the Greeks and Romans proscribed garlic in the temples (Moyers, 1996). Garlic was consumed largely by the working classes and avoided by the ruling classes and the wealthy (Moyers, 1996).

Garlic's popularity continued during the Middle Ages. Immigrants to the US took it there in the 1700s, but it rose in popularity only in the early 20th century. Traditionally, garlic is eaten raw, or in the juice, pulp, or paste form.

Medicine

There is extensive reference to its medicinal properties in both the Charakasamhita and the Sushrutasamhita, ancient Indian medical texts. Both Indians and Chinese regard garlic as an aphrodisiac. It aids digestion, improves respiration, and was used to get rid of intestinal worm infestation (Woodward, 1996). It helps in improving qi—life energy. Charakasamhita recommends the use of garlic to treat heart disease and arthritis too. Garlic's effect is also said to be diuretic.

The Ebers Papyrus (c. 1550 BC) prescribes the use of garlic in cases of high blood pressure and clogged arteries. Garlic was also prescribed to alleviate general malaise, and combat infestations of insects, worms, and parasites.

Hippocrates recommended the use of garlic in respiratory ailments, as a cleansing agent, and to treat abdominal growths. Dioscorides recommended the use of garlic to keep arteries clean. Pliny's Historica Naturalis mentions the use of garlic to improve digestion and to treat insect bites, arthritis, and convulsions.

Asian Herbs

Before the discovery of antibiotics, garlic was consumed in large quantities, especially during disease epidemics. Its anti-microbial properties were thought to provide protection. In 2002-2003, the SARS epidemic in China killed hundreds of people; garlic was consumed widely, hoping for protection against the virus.

It is a widely-researched species and is a popular herbal supplement cleared for use in the US, Europe, and across the globe. The plant is known to be effective in reducing high blood pressure, showing promise in reducing cardiovascular risk (Ackermann et al., 2001).

Garlic is useful in alleviating atherosclerosis (Berthold et al., 1998). It also tested positive for efficacy against Type 2 diabetes (Ashraf et al., 2005).

The antioxidant properties of aged garlic extract were observed by Dillon et al. (2003). Dorant et al. (1996) observed the spice's ability to moderate the impact of colorectal cancer. A similar correlation was made Durak et al. (2003) in prostate cancer patients. Heron et al. (1999) observed that garlic supplements can be used to treat parasitic infections.

Borelli et al. (2007) performed a study which reveals adverse interactions of garlic with certain drugs. Isonizid used to treat tuberculosis and in birth control pills, the cyclosporine given after organ transplant, and blood thinning medications could all be made less effective when garlic supplements are taken by patients.

Helicobacter pylori infects the stomachs of approximately 60% of the world's adult population (Cave, 1997). This number goes up to 95% in developing countries (Frenck and Clemens, 2003). This infection causes several gastric ailments that range from gastritis, duodenal and gastric ulcers, etc. (Dixon, 1992; and Nomura et al., 1994). O Gare et al. (2008) has studied the effects of garlic oil in a simulated gastric environment due to anti-Helibacter activity. The antibacterial effect on Helicobacter pylori stomach infections was observed by Salih et al. (2003). Both studies claim that garlic oil helped combat the infection.

The plant is rich in vitamins C and B6, magnesium, sodium, potassium, and calcium. The active ingredient isolated from the plant is allicin, along with a few other alkaloids. Allicin is responsible for the pungent odor of garlic.

Fresh garlic is said to be effective against bacteria like Escherichia coli, Salmonella enteritidis, and Staphylococcus aureus. It is topically used to treat fungal infections like ringworm, jock itch, athlete's foot, etc.

Homeopathy finds the plant useful too. It is part of the Bryonia group of medicine. The drug acts on the intestinal mucous membrane increasing peristalsis. It is used to treat colitis caused by pathological flora in the stomach, dyspepsia, and catarrhal affections. Homeopathy also uses the drug to treat atherosclerosis. The Bryonia group is used to treat tuberculosis.

In naturopathy, garlic is used for its anti-microbial and anti-fungal property and to treat intestinal worms, fungal infections, etc. Native American tribes and other folkloric medical systems use garlic to treat cold, chest, and lung infections.

Production and Trade

The global production of garlic, according to FAOSTAT (Food and Agriculture Organization Statistics) 2013 data was put at 24.255 million metric tons. China is the preeminent producer with 19.234 million metric tons, followed by India. India produces only a fraction of China's produce at 1.259 million metric tons. The US production is small at 175,000 metric tons. The total acreage of garlic worldwide is around 1.5 million hectares.

California accounts for nearly the whole of US garlic production. Gilroy is the center for local garlic processing, packaging, and shipping. US imports small quantities of garlic from China, Canada, Mexico, and Argentina. FAS 2011 figures for fresh garlic import stand at 74,531 metric tons. Dried garlic import was an additional 30,170 metric tons.

There are frequent complaints about the quality of the garlic from China in the global market. Anti-dumping duties have been levied on imports of Chinese garlic by both the EU and the US but has failed in checking this practice. Fermented garlic, black in color, is also consumed. It forms, though, just about 1% of the garlic consumed in the US.

Per capita consumption of garlic in the US has been put at two pounds per year (Agriculture Marketing Resource Center 2014).

Onion not just vegetable but also medicine

In traditional Chinese medicine, onion is yang food. In Ayurveda too, onion is said to stimulate the human body. Before the arrival of European settlers in the US, Native Americans were known to consume wild onion as a vegetable and use it for seasoning food. Allium sibiricum and Allium validum were two prominent wild species in North America. A. sibiricum is also found in the UK where it is referred to as wild garlic.

Wild onion was used to accord relief in cold, cough, asthma, etc. Both wild and the cultivated species help expel gas and calm an upset stomach. The general morphology and the flower pattern in the wild and cultivated varieties are similar.

It is a perennial plant. It is replanted two or more times a year. If left un-harvested, the green shoots shrivel up and the plant hibernates for the winter. It sprouts back in the spring when climatic conditions become conducive for growth. The height of the average plant ranges between one to two feet

A flowering shoot emanates straight from the bulb buried in the ground. The onion bulbs are harvested just before the onset of flowering. Usually, there is a single bulb to a plant, but some may grow multiple bulbs too. In trade, these differentiated as shallots and potato onions.

Onion has been used as both food and medicine since ancient times. Egyptians, Chinese, Indians, Romans, Greeks, and the tribal societies of Latin and North America were all familiar with this plant. There is mention of the plant in both the orally transmitted lore of ancient times as well as in written literature. The plant has been in cultivation for at least over 3,000 years. A. cepa is the cultivated variety of Allium genus.

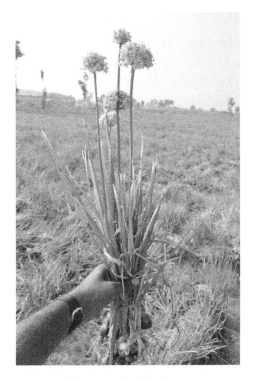

Picture 22: Allium cepa
Photo: Dr Ravikumar, Senior botanist, FRLHT

Along with garlic, onion was a staple food of the Egyptian pyramid builders. It was an ancient belief that consuming onions gave strength to the body. In ancient Greece and Rome, onion was fed to athletes and gladiators

The Egyptians believed that the many layers of onion that are arranged in concentric spheres represent eternal life and included onion in their funeral

The white variety is sharper and more pungent in flavor. Red onions have a milder flavor.

There is yet another very mild variety called the sweet onion. This variety of onion perishes faster in comparison to the others. Sweet onions are thinly sliced and served in salads. They are mainly used to garnish food. Pungency of the onion can be reduced by soaking them in water after slicing.

Buddhists and Jains, even today, proscribe the consumption of onion.[28] The Taoist sage Tsang Tsze said that garlic and onion have detrimental effects on the liver, spleen, lungs, kidneys, and heart, but there is little support in modern science for these views.

Medicine

In traditional Chinese medicine, onions are said to enhance chi or energy. They induce urination and perspiration. It is recommended for consumption when the weather is cold. Mixed with garlic and sugar, onion is said to ameliorate respiratory stress induced by cold weather.

Herbal medicine systems of both China and India regard onion to be beneficial to the cardiovascular system. It helps reduce blood platelet aggregation and cholesterol levels. Onion, both ripe and green, are said to help improve digestion. They also keep oral bacteria under check.

Shallots have higher phenolic content and high levels of antioxidants. These antioxidants are preserved if cooked in low heat. Onions are also anti-inflammatory and can help reduce arthritic and associated pains in bones and joints.

Both Chinese and traditional Indian herbal medicine systems claim that onion and its seed enhance libido. Hot water extract of onion is said to

---

28   Ayurveda regards onions and garlic as tamasic food.

be an aphrodisiac for both men and women. Onion is used to treat colds, improve digestion, heart ailments, blisters, boils, and topical scars. Fresh onion is consumed to ameliorate amenorrhea, menstrual, and uterine pains.

Mixed with Adhatoda vasica and honey, onion is recommended as a treatment for tuberculosis. Unani and Ayurveda doctors use onion in dried, roasted, fresh, and juice forms to treat respiratory, gastric, eye diseases, and diabetes.

Kumar et al. (2010) recommends use of fresh onion extracts in coughs, colds, and other respiratory ailments. WHO (World Health Organization) supports the use of onions to treat appetite loss and prevent atherosclerosis (hardening of arteries).

In homeopathy, Allium cepa is recommended in cases of flu and gastrointestinal ailments. Onion and garlic are rich in sulphur compounds. They possess anti-diabetic, antibiotic, hyocholesterolemic, fibrinolytic properties (Augusti, 1996).

Allium cepa extract was shown to have anti-microbial action against Staphylococcus aureus bacteria (Eltaweel, 2013). Experiments done by Azu et al. (2006) demonstrated anti-microbial properties of onion and ginger extracts against other bacteria like Escherichia coli, Salmonella typhi (causes typhoid), and Bacillus subtillis.

The anti-cancer property of onion has been studied by Votto et al. (2010). Their experiments showed that cell death occurs when exposed to onion extract, due to damage caused to the DNA.

A randomized, controlled, single blind study revealed that eight weeks of application of a proprietary onion extract gel (once a day) led to significant reduction of scar tissue in patients. Animal trials have validated anti-diabetic properties of the plant (Jevas, 2011).

The German Federal Health Agency's Commission has approved onion as an antibacterial agent. The Commission has concluded that onion is a healthful vegetable that may have many medical benefits.

While onion is found to be beneficial to humans, it was observed to be harmful to animals like cats, dogs, sheep, and goats. Animals fed a diet rich in onions can turn anemic with impaired oxygen transport (American Society of Prevention of Cruelty to Animals).

The plant is rich in antioxidants, flavonoids, and phenolic compounds. The strong smell emanating from the onion is attributed to cysteine sulphoxide.

GINGER and their little known medicinal properties

Ginger, the underground rhizome of Zingiber officinale plant, is a spice popular throughout the world. The plant's probable origin is in India, although the species is referred to in ancient Chinese works too. Probably, the warmer southern regions of China and northern parts of India were the original home of ginger. Ginger is integral to Chinese cuisine and popular in Indian food too.

The cuneiform scrolls from King Ashurbanipal of Assyria period (668-633 BC) make a mention of aromatic plants. Ginger, along other spices like saffron and cumin, are mentioned therein. King Merodach-baladan II(721-710 BC) has recorded that ginger was one of the aromatic plants that were grown in the imperial gardens of Babylonia. Records from the time of King Cyrus (559-529 BC) note a large purchase of 395,000 bunches of ginger.

There are references to the use of ginger as medicine in writings of Dioscorides[29] who mentions it in his Materia Medica, written between

---

29   Pedanus Dioscorides was a physician who traveled the Roman Empire with Emperor Nero's army. He had a passion for local herbs and collected these from wherever he traveled. He published in five volumes a treatise on herbs in 70 AD. This was called De Materia Medica. This work was later supplemented with works of other authors from India, Middle East, and Europe.

50 AD and 70 AD. Dioscorides lived during the reign of the Roman Emperor Nero. He describes the action of ginger. Ginger is also referred to in the Ebers Papyrus of Egypt (c. 1550 BC). All ancient herbal medical systems, like the Chinese, Ayurvedic, Greek, and Egyptian, refer to the use of ginger as a digestive aid

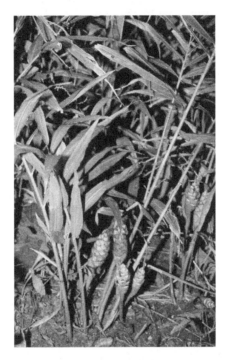

Picture 23 Zingiber officinale plants
Photo: Dr Ravikumar, Senior botanist, FRLHT

The practice of using ginger spread from Asia to the rest of the world through trade. The Romans were major importers of spices, for which they paid in gold. Ginger was one of the many Asian spices imported into Southern Europe. As the empire of Rome extended to North Africa, Turkey, Persia, and Western Europe, the use of ginger as medicine and in food became more and more widespread.

Marco Polo refers to use of ginger in food in China in the 12th century AD.

With the rise of the European powers, and the colonization of Asia and North America, ginger producing areas lost control of trade. Colonization also spread the use of ginger to North and Latin America.

Romans were known to use spices including ginger to flavor their wines, healing oils, and food. Spices were expensive, and consumption was largely confined to the rich classes of Rome. The practice of using ginger to flavor wines continued in Europe through the Middle Ages. Most Asians consume ginger fresh as it intensifies the flavor. Dried ginger is not preferred in Chinese cuisine.

The trade in ginger from ancient to medieval times was largely in the dried or the powder form. Ginger plants were also carried in pots in trader boats, mainly for consumption by the traders and the crew. Mature ginger rhizomes can be preserved for over a month and are also traded.

Ginger was believed to be effective against scurvy. With modern medical knowledge, this belief has been proven wrong as scurvy is caused by a deficiency of vitamin C, and ginger is not a source of this vitamin.

South Asians who were brought to the Caribbean as indentured labor brought ginger with them. The plant quickly acclimatized to the soil and the environment of the islands. It was soon indigenized and became a popular crop of these islands. Today, ginger is grown throughout the tropics. In the 20thcentury, ginger became very popular in the US where it was used as a digestive aid. It was also a preferred ingredient in the diet of Revolutionary soldiers during the Civil War.

Ginger (Zingier officinale) belongs to the same family (Zingiberaceae) as other popular Asian spices like turmeric, cardamom, and galangal. It is an herbaceous perennial plant. The modified shoot, the rhizome, acts as an underground plant anchor and is the portion used as the spice.

The herb rarely grows beyond one meter in height. The plant bears beautiful flowers. The rhizome is fibrous and covered with a brown skin, which is removed before use. When not fully ripe, it has a pinkish hue. Its aroma is the highest when still young. However, it rots quickly at this stage and must be consumed within a week.

India and China are the largest producers of ginger in the world producing 703,000 and 425,000 metric tons of ginger respectively (Food and Agricultural Organization, 2012 data). Other major producers are Nepal, followed by Nigeria, Thailand, and Indonesia. Together, these six countries produced 2.095 million metric tons of ginger rhizome in 2012 (FAO, 2012 data).

Food

Ginger in Asia is used in soups, curries, stews, and meats. It is pickled with lemon and vinegar and eaten as a spicy accompaniment. Mature ginger is fibrous and has no juice. Immature rhizomes are pink, juicy, and more aromatic in comparison.

Much of pickle preserves made in India and China are made from the immature ginger rhizomes. In India, mature ginger is sliced and mixed with brown sugar syrup, tamarind, other spices, and dry fruits to make a delicious syrupy candy.

In Europe, ginger was added to buttermilk drinks and in bread. Ginger bread became popular in England during the reign of Queen Elizabeth I. Ginger flavored cookies, breads, and other bakes are popular across the globe.

Ginger can be stored for a whole season and lasts up to six months when packed in an airtight plastic bag and refrigerated. Unpeeled mature ginger rhizomes can be stored outside for up to a month and still be fit for consumption. Before the days of the refrigerator, ginger rhizomes were often stored in a sand pit.

During the Sui Dynasty (581-619 AD) in China, tea became a popular refreshing drink, often infused with salt, spices, ginger, and orange peel. Ginger tea is brewed with grated or minced fresh ginger. The decoction can be mixed with honey and lemon and is popular amongst tea drinkers. Another popular ginger tea combination is with peppermint, sugar, and milk. The drink has a zingy flavor.

Medicine

In India, a tea decoction with ginger, pepper, sugar, and milk is a common home remedy for relief from cold. Ginger tea is, however, not recommended to people who have dry cough or are suffering from dehydration. Ginger is said to possess expectorant properties and is also a digestive aid. Ginger tea is advised to prevent motion sickness. This tea helps reduce heartburn and calms an upset stomach and mind. It is recommended in cold and flu conditions and has anti-inflammatory properties.

The Chinese believe that the spice can help neutralize poisons in food. Dioscorides also regarded ginger as an antidote to poison. In traditional Chinese medicine, ginger is prescribed for relief from arthritis-induced pain, discomfort from cramps, bloating during menstruation, and liver ailments. Ginger tea is used to improve circulation and to flush out toxins and poisons from the body.

Chinese herbalists also say that the spice is useful in preventing heart disease and gives a boost to the immune system. Ginger tea is regarded as an aphrodisiac. Drinking a cup of ginger tea, a day is supposed to raise sperm mobility and count. Ginger tea is caffeine-free and is regarded as a health drink. Many of the medicinal uses as per traditional Chinese medicine are recommended in Ayurveda too.

An oil is distilled from the rhizome of ginger through steam distilling it. This pale to dark colored oil is very aromatic, peppery, and camphor-like with a lemon note. Mixed with citrus and other fruity flavors, ginger is used in perfumery.

Essential oil of ginger should not be directly administered on the skin as this could cause a rash. The principal constituents of the oil include a range of sesquiterpenes, sesquiterpenic alcohols, and terpenes along with citrol and resins.

Its medicinal properties are like that of the ginger rhizome. However, ginger and its oil may increase risk in people susceptible of bleeding disorders. This could be due to the anti-coagulant property of the spice (Srivastava et al., 1984). Ginger is said to lower blood sugar.

The study of the pharmacological actions of ginger and compounds isolated therefrom found it a safe herbal medicine with only a few side effects. The action of the ginger compounds was immune-modulatory, anti-tumorigenic, anti-inflammatory, anti-apoptotic, anti-hyperglycemic, anti-lipidemic, and anti-emetic. They state that further studies are required to understand the effect of consumption over long periods of time.

Trials with highly purified ginger extract were conducted by Altman et al. (2011) on patients with osteoarthritis pain caused by standing for extended periods of time. The relief observed was moderate with mild gastrointestinal side effects.

Another randomized, placebo-controlled crossover study was conducted to study the impact of ginger extracts and ibuprofen in patients suffering from the pain of osteoarthritis. It was observed that there was not much variation between the control and active groups during the first three months of the study. However, at the end of six months, the active group showed significantly superior results over the placebo group (Bliddal et al., 2000)., These studies appear to validate the beneficial impact of ginger on osteoarthritis patients as mentioned in ancient Chinese and Ayurvedic herbal medicine practices. Ginger and turmeric are used as herbal remedies for osteoarthritis. (Wigler et al., 2003)

Another traditional medicinal use of ginger was with its anti-nausea properties. Apariman et al. from the Thai Medical Association (2006) showed that ginger was effective in preventing nausea. It had borderline significance in preventing vomiting after a gynecological laparoscopy six hours post-operation.

Another post-operative trial aimed at determining anti-emetic impact of ginger extract was conducted on 60 women. It was found that the incidence of nausea was reduced in the group that was administered ginger extract when compared with the placebo group (Bone et al., 1990).

However, another trial conducted on 180 women to test the postoperative anti-emetic impact of ginger indicated no impact of ginger on the patients (Eberhart et al., 2003). Positive results were also observed by a study on post-operative patients by Pongropaw et al. (2007). Opposing results that indicated positive anti-emetic effect of ginger were observed in other studies (Chaiyakunapruk, 2006).

Ginger was given in the dry powdered form to post-operative Caesarian section patients. It was observed that while the number of nausea episodes did get reduced, it had no effective impact on incidence of nausea, vomiting, or pain (Kalava et al., 2013). Another study reported by Zeraati et al. (2016) on patients who underwent ceasarian operation and had been subjected to spinal anaesthesia, too, shows that severity of nausea was reduced with ginger extracts. Reviews of studies to assess the impact of ginger on travel-related motion sickness was conducted by Langner et al. (1999), and they conclude that the herb did reduce incidence of travel-related motion sickness. Another study also supports the anti-nausea property of ginger too.

The effect of ginger on blood platelet aggregation in coronary heart disease patients was studied. It was observed that a single dose of 10 grams of powdered ginger produced a significant reduction on platelet aggregation (Bordia et al., 1997). However, they observed that ginger did not affect blood lipids and blood sugar.

Ginger extract consumed by mice affected by atherosclerosis resulted in reduction of lesions (Fuhrman et al., 2000). The anti-platelet effect of ginger compounds and their derivatives were observed to be better than that of the known anti-platelet medicine aspirin (Nurtjahja-Tjendraptra et al., 2003).

Ginger was also found to help lower cholesterol, clotting of blood and inflammations (Thomson et al., 2002). 6 Gingerol is a natural product of ginger. Experiments with it have shown that it has anti-tumor and anti-cancer properties (Lee et al., 2008). The anti-cancer properties were further studied, and the results show its beneficial effect in human leukemia cells (Wang et al., 2003).

The effect of gingerols on Helicobacter pylori bacteria that cause gastritis and cancer in the stomach was studied and results indicate that the herb has chemo preventive effects (Mahady et al., 2003). However, studies that observed ginger's anti-coagulating properties have been inconclusive (Vaes et al., 2000).

Star anise a cure for bird flu

Star anise is one of the ingredients in the Chinese five-spice powder. It is the dried star-shaped fruit pods of the mid-sized evergreen Illicium verum tree. The tree belongs to Schisandraceae family. Star anise is different from anise (Pimpinella anisum) which is from the parsley family (Apiaceae). The tree is a native of Southwest China and Northeast Vietnam. It is also found in the state of Arunachal Pradesh in India,

Laos, Philippines, and Jamaica. Both star anise and anise yield anethole, an essential oil. Both spices are used to flavor drinks and confectionary.

The tree is not found in the wild now. It prefers woodlands and a bit of shade and tolerates low temperature down to -10 degrees Celsius. According to kew. org the plant has been under cultivation since 2000 BC. It probably existed in the wild across the Southeast Asian region.

The tree bears scented flowers and is of ornamental quality too. The wood is fragrant and is used in construction and furniture making. The tree is cultivated as an intercrop with mandarin orange or tea. It is also cultivated in pure stands. It is a preferred agroforestry species for plant growers as it gives them a reasonable rate of return.

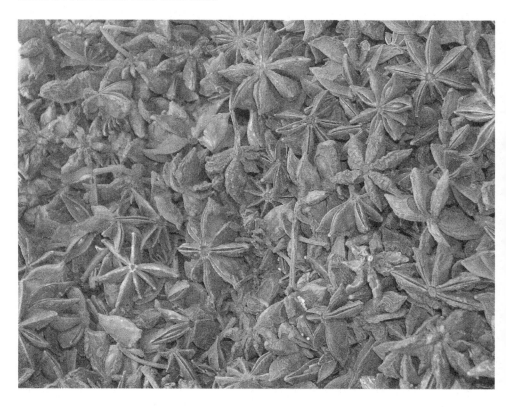

Picture 24 Star anise spice
Photo: Dr Ravikumar, Senior botanist, FRLHT

The Chinese star anise should be distinguished from the Japanese star anise which is a different species—Illicium anisatum. The Japanese species is highly toxic. Sometimes Chinese star anise tea products are adulterated with Japanese star anise and are unsafe to human health. Once in powder form, it is difficult to tell the difference by just looking at them. The toxicity of the Japanese star anise is due to the presence of sikimitoxin.

Star anise was used as a carminative for infants. After several infants in Spain were observed to suffer serious gastrointestinal and neurological symptoms, the causes were sought to be examined. It was suspected that this was a case of adulteration. Fernandez et al. studied 23 cases. The study confirmed that these symptoms were due to contamination of Chinese star anise (Illicium verum) with the toxic Japanese star anise— Illicium anisatum (Fernandez et al., 2002). The neurotoxicity symptom in infants caused from the toxic effect of Illicium anisatum was further confirmed by a study conducted by Ludlow et al. (2004).

The US FDA in 2003 issued an advisory regarding consumption of star anise tea. Tea contaminated with the Japanese anise is suspected to cause neurological symptoms. However, star anise as a spice has been given the Generally Recognized as Safe (GRAS) certificate by the US FDA. Some believe that these spicy teas are beneficial and may help in indigestion, but others associate it with seizures, vomiting, and agitative behavior.

Whole Chinese star anise is used not just in cuisine but also in soups and teas in China and Southeast Asia. It is also used to flavor baked dishes. It gives a licorice flavor to dishes and is a popular spice in pork and poultry food. It is used both as whole and in the ground form.

Thai iced tea which is brewed from black tea is often flavored with star anise powder, cinnamon, licorice, vanilla, and orange flowers. In India, the spice is sometimes added as an ingredient of garam masala, a spice mix used across South Asia, Persia, and Indonesia.

Star anise is not related to the common anise Anisum vulgare. The species was first introduced in Europe in the 16th century. Both Chinese star anise and regular anise seed contain the compound anethole, giving the two species a nearly identical flavor, which is strong, sweet, and smells like licorice. In Europe and the US, the spice is used to flavor fruit compotes, jams, and liqueurs. The flavor of this spice has resemblance to fennel and basil and is used as a substitute to anise.

The fruit is harvested before it matures and dried to produce the spice. The fruit pod is a five- to eight-pointed star, and the size is rarely more than an inch and a half in length. The flavor of star anise is more bitter when compared to the anise seed. The stars are available as whole and are ground into a powder form.

Most of the star anise is produced from trees growing in Chinese provinces of Guangxi and Yunnan. In Guangxi province, it is estimated that 350,000 hectares of farmland is devoted to star anise tree farming. The annual production from this area has been put at 80,000 metric tons. The commercial harvesting of the fruit from these trees starts from the sixth year onward.

Essential Oil

The essential oil is produced by steam extracting fresh and partly dried fruits. The oil is clear and colorless to pale yellow. It is aromatic and has a sweet and pleasant fragrance like that of anise. It is said to relax, improve sleep patterns, and reduce tiredness. The oil blends well with bay, cardamom, coriander, dill, cedarwood orange, and other natural oils. Being highly fragrant, it's used in cooking, perfumery, soaps, toothpastes, mouthwashes, and skin creams. The Japanese star anise, which is highly toxic, is burnt for its fragrance.

Medicinal Use

However, 90% of star anise crop is used to extract shikimic acid, a chemical ingredient of the bird flu vaccine oseltamivir, most commonly known as Tamiflu.

With China producing most of the star anise in the world, prices of the spice rose dramatically during the bird flu epidemic of the early 21st century. The demand for the vaccine was huge, and research for a chemical variant of shikimic acid was successful. These have been since patented.

In traditional Chinese medicine, star anise is regarded to be useful in relieving ailments related to cold. The spice is prescribed to aid digestion, promote health of female reproductive organs, improve lactation in mothers, in cough mixtures, as a diuretic, antibacterial, anti-fungal medicine, and to alleviate respiratory ailments. The species is also used in natural breath fresheners. A compound linalool present in the spice contains antioxidant properties.

Comparison with insecticidal compounds like detamethrin and hydramethylnon found that Illium verum (star anise) is a naturally occurring insect control agent that is rich in anethole molecules. The experiments revealed that the naturally occurring agents were useful to contain
populations of Blattella germanica, a German cockroach species. The anti-microbial properties are evident; anethole isolated from the dried fruit of star anise was observed to be potent against bacteria, yeast, and fungal strains too (De et al., 2002).

Sichuan pepper a culinary spice that tingles and numbs at the same time

Sichuan peppercorn is one of the spices in the five-spice powder popular in Chinese cuisine. It comes from the outer peel of a berry fruit and is locally known as "huajiao." The earliest references to Sichuan pepper, also called Schezuan pepper, are seen in the Classic of Poetry, said to have been compiled by Confucius (551-479 BC).

Sichuan pepper comes from several species of Zanthoxylum. These species are distributed across China, Nepal, Bhutan, Japan, Korea, Indonesia, and India. An allied species, Zanthoxylum americanum, is found in North America.

The genus Zanthoxylum belongs to the family Rutaceae. Orange also belongs to Rutaceae. Zanthoxylum simulans, Z. bungeanum, Z. planispinum, and Z. armatum are some of the common sources of Sichuan pepper. Z. bungeanum is valued most in traditional Chinese medicine. Z. armatum is found in the

Himalayan region and parts of South and East Asia, Z. avicennae in Indonesia, and Z. piperitum in Central and East China, Japan, and Korea.

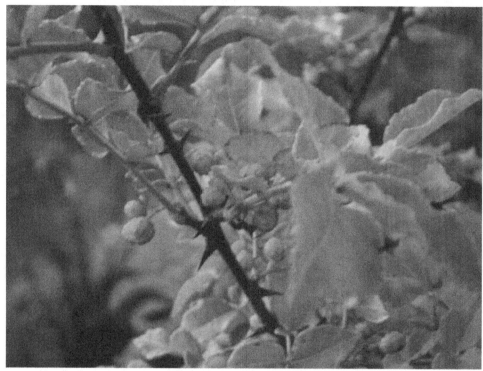

Picture 25 Sichuan pepper plants in China
Photo by: Vmenkov

Z. americanum is a North American species, colloquially called the toothache tree because of its anesthetic properties that were used by the Native Americans to relieve a toothache. Unripe fruits and wood of the young shoots were chewed for that purpose.

The pepper was used in China as a medicinal herb and for seasoning food. In ancient China, the pepper was steeped in wine to give it a unique peppery lemony flavor. Avicenna (c. 1020 AD) referred to the spice as fagara. The spice came to the Persian and Arabic region with traders who, taking the Silk

Route, came from China to the region. Sichuan pepper crop is a popular agro-forestry non-timber forest product. Harvesting of the berries is done when the fruit is ripe, as early harvesting exposes it to fungal infections and renders the production unusable.

The Sichuan pepper tree bears small reddish-brown berries which when split open release round black seeds. The texture of the seeds is like sand and is discarded. It is the outer coat of the berry that is dried and used as a spice. Whole berries or as ground into powder can be also used as a spice.

The pungency of Sichuan pepper comes from pungent alkamides stored in the pericarp. Alkamides are absent in the seeds. The lack of standardization and absence of collection, storage and logistics protocols in collection, and processing has often led to health concerns being raised by the major spice importing countries of Europe and the US.

Import of Sichuan pepper was banned in the US in 2005 to protect the orange crop that could be destroyed from citrus canker disease that had infected peppercorns. Untreated berries carrying the bacteria Xanthomonas axonopodiscan have a disastrous effect on citrus crops.

Bacteria contained in Sichuan pepper is killed when berries are gently roasted, a traditional practice. Imports into the US were re-opened but only for heat-treated peppercorns. Limited quantities of Chinese peppers are imported into the US mainly for consumption by Chinese eateries and lovers of Chinese food.

Sichuan pepper, known locally as timur in Nepal, is exported mainly to India. In Nepal the spice trees are cultivated as an agro-forestry species. The crop is raised on degraded forest and non-forest sites in the country. It is estimated that Nepal annually exports 850 to 1,100 metric tons of this spice to India, mostly raw.

Food

Oil infused with roasted peppercorns and mixed with salt and other

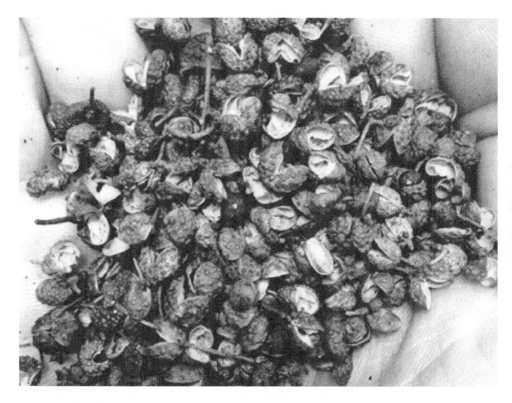

Picture 26: Sichuan peppercorns
Photo: Max Ronnersjo

condiments is popular in Chinese and East Asian cuisine. Some of this oil-based peppercorn product is exported to France, Italy, and other West European countries. Leaves of these trees are also used to flavor food in China.

Different species of Zanthoxylum have their own distinct flavor. Z. alatum is spicy, and Z. avicennae and Z. schinifolium are anise-like in flavor. Most species have a lemon-like odor with warm and woodsy overtones. Z.

piperitumleaves have a fresh flavor that lies somewhere in between the mint and the lime.

The Korean species Z. schinifolium has aromatic seeds and both the pericarp (outer part of the berry) and seed are used. The spice gives a tingling, numbing sensation to the mouth which is different from the hot taste you get when you eat chilly or black pepper. Z. schinifolium is only pungent, an exception from the typical numbing sensation quality of other species.

Sichuan pepper is known in trade by multiple names—Szechuan pepper, Chinese pepper, Japanese pepper, aniseed pepper, Chinese prickly-ash, fagara, sansho, Nepal pepper or timur, Indonesian lemon pepper, etc. The spice is extensively used in cuisine of China, Southeast Asian countries, Tibet, Nepal, and India. It is sometimes added to garam masala too.

Sichuan pepper spice is popular in those regions where the food is preferred hot and spicy like in Sichuan or Szechuan province, Thailand, and other parts of the world. This spice is used in Ma La sauce (mala literally means "numbing and spicy") which describes the effect of the spice on the palate. The spice is also used in Sichuan cakes and biscuits.

The spice is used in rice, noodles, momos, thupkas, vegetables, meat, fowl, and pork. In Indonesian Batak cuisine, its ground and mixed with chilis to make a paste and eaten as an accompaniment with grilled pork, carp, and other dishes. The spice aids digestion by increased release of gastro intestinal juice and enzymes. However, it is also known to cause stomach upset, irritation, and exasperate peptic ulcers. Sichuan pepper is therefore best consumed in moderation.

Medicine

In traditional Chinese medicine, Sichuan pepper is said to relieve pain, kill parasites, and relieve itching. It is used to treat gastro-intestinal ailments and infections of the stomach. It has anti-septic, anti-spasmodic, carminative, expectorant, and stimulant properties.

Nepalese use powder from timur seeds (timur is the local name of Sichuan pepper species found in the country) to detach leeches, a common menace in moist tropics, from the body. It is also regarded to be a disinfectant.

It is said to be analgesic, anti-convulsant, anti-helminthic, anti-inflammatory, anti-microbial, anti-parasitic, anti-platelet, and gastroprotective. The antioxidant property is said to protect the body against cancer and diabetes. The analgesic activity of the root bark of Zanthoxylum xanthozyloides is attributed to the spice's ability to inhibit prostaglandin production (Prempeh et al., 2008).

The anti-inflammatory and analgesic activity of leaves and stem bark of Zanthoxylum riedelianum was observed on experimental mice (Lima et al., 2007). Anti-inflammatory properties of Z. nitidum and Z. armatum were validated in experiments conducted on mice (Gou et al., 2011).

The antioxidant properties of Zanthoxylum alatum (the variety popular in Pakistan) were validated in experiments on the brain, kidney, and liver of rats. (Batool et al., 2010). The presence of antioxidants in Japanese pepper fruit (Zanthoxylum piperita) was seen in studies by Japanese scientists (Histamoi et al., 2000). Glycoprotein of Zanthoxylum piperitum was observed to have a hepatoprotective effect. This property was associated to the species antioxidative action (Lee et al., 2008).

Toothpaste containing Z. nitidum showed decrease in incidence of dental plaque and enhanced gingival health (Wan et al., 2005). As has been mentioned earlier, Native Americans used Z. americanum to ameliorate toothache.

An essential oil from the leaves and fruits of Z. leprieurii, Z. macrophylla, and Z. xanthoxyloides from the Cameroon is extracted by hydrodistillation. The anti-inflammatory and antioxidant property of these oils was also observed (Dongmo et al., 2008).

The anti-fungal action of Z. armatum against Bipolaris sorokiniana, an important leaf blight pathogen of wheat, was studied. The essential oil of Z. armatum showed inhibition of fungal mycelia when exposed to higher concentrations of 40 ml (Manandhar et al., 2005). The anti-fungal properties of Z. americanum was observed in experiments (Bafi-Yeboa et al., 2005). The anti-helminthic property of seeds of Z. armatum against the helminth worm Pheretima posthuma was also observed (Mehta et al., 2012).

Ethanolic extracts of Zanthoxylum gilletii, Funtumia elastic, and Rauvolfia vomitoria were tested on isolates gathered from malaria (Plasmodium falciparum) patients who came for consultation at the National Institute of Public Health in Abidjan (Cote-d'Ivoire). The results showed that the extracts exhibited strong anti-malarial action (Zirihi et al., 2009).

Experiments to test the anti-convulsant property of Zanthoxylum capenseshowed that seizures were delayed after administration of methanol leaf extracts on experimental mice (Amabeoku et al., 2010).

Fennel an after meal digestive

Fennel probably originated in the Mediterranean region. Its use in Chinese cuisine and medicine started only during the Tang Dynasty (c. 618-907 AD). There are references to fennel in the Tang Dynasty Materia Media. It is an ingredient in the five-spice powder used extensively to flavor Chinese cuisine. It could be that the spice was being imported into China via the Silk Route.

The Greek name for fennel is marathon, a place where in a field of fennel in 490 BC a battle was fought between the Persians and the Greeks. According to Greek mythology, knowledge came to man from Mount Olympus in the form of a fiery coal contained in a fennel stalk (Encyclopedia Britannica), a source of strength and courage. Both the Ancient Greeks and Romans used fennel in their cuisine and medicine.

Pliny refers to its use in medicine in his Naturalis Historia (23-79 AD). The

Ancient Egyptians believed that plaque on teeth can be prevented by consuming a mixture of fennel seeds and barberry. In the Middle Ages, Europeans and Chinese hung stalks of fennel at the doorway to keep evil away.

Foeniculum vulgare is the botanical name of fennel. It belongs to the carrot family (Umbelliferae syn Apiaceae). Some other popular species from this family includes anise seed, carrot, coriander, dill,

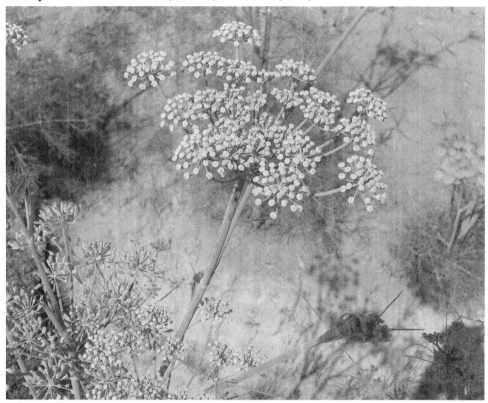

Picture 27 Fennel plant in flower
Photo by: Sudhir Ahluwalia

and parsley. The plant is grown extensively in the dry ecosystems of the Mediterranean shoreline. Fennel, today, is cultivated throughout Southern Europe, Southern China, US, France, India, and Russia.

Fennel is not frost hardy, but it prefers cool weather. The underground bulb takes around three months to form. Foeniculum vulgare, some claim, has two sub-species, piperitum and vulgare. The seeds of piperitum are bitter. The seeds of the vulgare sub-species are sweet. Morphological differences between the two sub-species are not defined. Dozens of varieties of fennel have been identified.

It is a perennial with aromatic feathery leaves. It bears yellow flowers arranged in the form of a bouquet or umbel. The flower petals, after they are dried, expose a cluster of seeds that are picked and dried for use. The dried seed is green and splits in half when ripe.

Fennel inhibits the growth of other vegetable crops like beans, tomatoes, etc. and can only be cultivated as a pure crop. Its growth too is inhibited by species like coriander and wormwood. The plant flowers profusely and is a magnet to bees and flies. When grown with other crops, pests get attracted to fennel, protecting the main crop.

Dill and fennel come from the same family. They are also known to cross-fertilize. Cross-fertilization leads to a change of flavor, and care should be taken to grow these crops side by side. The plant propagates well by seed and has become an invasive weed in exotic locations like those of Australia and the US. It usually grows to six feet in height.

Food

It is a familiar cooking herb in the Mediterranean and is popular in the whole belt from Greece to Egypt. Ancient Romans cultivated fennel for its aromatic seeds and edible shoots. Ancient Egyptians too used fennel both in food and as medicine. There are references to fennel in the Anglo-Saxon cuisine. Charlemagne's (8th century AD) imperial farms had fennel crops too.

Fennel seed is sweet and is eaten as a mouth freshener. It is a popular after-meal digestive in India. The Chinese use the leaves and stems in their cooking with the seeds added as spice. The young, tender leaves are used to garnish food, as a salad, to flavor soups, sauces, desserts, and absinthe. Herbal tea can be infused with fennel. It is used as flavor in natural toothpastes. The bulb and shoots have a mild crunchy texture and sweet flavor.

All parts of the plant from the bulb to the seed are edible. When grown as a vegetable, the flowering stalks are sniped off to prevent diversion of nutrients into flowering and seeding. The vegetable is eaten both cooked and raw. The leaves and seed of fennel taste like the aniseed flavor because of the anethole. In the US, it is sometimes mislabeled as anise.

A review of the Food and Agriculture Organization 2008 data tells us that the production of anise, star anise, fennel, and coriander is the highest in India. Annual production is placed at 110,000 metric tons. Other major producers are Mexico with 49,688 MT, China with 40,000 MT, and Iran with 30,000 MT.

Fennel production in the US is limited to a few thousand acres of crop in California, and most of the fennel consumed is imported from India, Mexico, and Egypt. In India, most of its production is limited to Gujarat, Uttar Pradesh, and Rajasthan. According to Spices Board of India, 7,250 MT of fennel was exported from India in 2010-11, most of it was to the Middle East and some to the US. The per-hectare yields vary from 1,500 to 1,800 kilograms. Most cultivation is done for its seed. Fennel seed is placed in the GRAS (Generally Recognized as Safe) category by the US FDA.

Fennel Oil

The seed can yield up to 5% of a clear-colored essential oil. The flavor of the oil is due to fenchone and anethole. Fenchone is bitter tasting and anethole has a sweet anise-like flavor. It is the proportion of the two molecules that determines taste and flavor of a variety.

Plants growing in the Mediterranean region generally have sweeter oil while those in Northern and Central Europe are bitter. A well-dried and fully-ripened seed yields much sweeter and more fragrant oil.

Fennel oil is used in fragrances and blends well with oil of sandalwood, lavender, geranium, and rose. The anti-aging effect of a cream that contained 4% fennel extract was studied, and results validated the anti-aging property of the spice extract (Rasul et al., 2012).

It is also seen to possess a range of medicinal properties that are comparable to the seed and other parts of the plant. However, skin allergies are known to occur when the oil is in direct contact with the skin. Ingestion of the oil can cause vomiting and pulmonary edema.

The essential oil of fennel helped reduce microbial activity of disease-causing microorganisms like Staphylococcus aureus, Candida albicans, Bacillus aureus, and Aspergillus flavus (Roby et al., 2013). Numerous other studies have validated the antibacterial properties of fennel (Kaur et al., 2009; Manonmani et al., 2011; and Kazem et al., 2012).

A coumarin molecule responsible the anti-mycobacterial property has been isolated (Esquivel-Ferrino et al., 2012). The anti-fungal properties of fennel essential oils have also been validated (Park et al., 2010; and Thakur et al., 2013).

Fennel essential oil can control house mites and was observed to be comparable to the commercial repellent benzyl benzoate (Lee, 2004). Its larvicidal ability against mosquito Anopheles stephensi was also observed (Sedhaghat et al., 2011).

Fennel essential oil helped reduce dysmenorrhea (menstrual pain) symptoms in studies conducted on rats (Ostad et al., 2001). Studies have shown fennel essential oil reducing abnormal sperm in mice.

The anti-diabetic property of essential oil of fennel was observed in experiments on rats (EL-Soud et al., 2011). Fennel essential oil was seen to reduce toxicity in the liver in experiments conducted on rats (Ozbek et al., 2003).

The anti-platelet property of anethole molecule contained in the Foeniculum vulgare essential oil was studied. The experiments showed that the essential oil can possess clot destabilization property and a vasorelaxant action (Tognolini et al., 2007). The blood pressure reducing properties were also observed (Abdul-Ghani et al., 1988; and El Bardai et al., 2001).

Medicine

In Chinese medicine, fennel is believed to strengthen eyesight, relieve cough, assist in digestion, treat stomach ailments, menstrual, and
respiratory disorders. A poultice made from fennel was externally applied as a remedy for snake and scorpion bites. The Chinese believe that fennel brings balance to qi. Fennel was used in traditional Chinese medicine as a laxative, to treat cold, and to treat liver, kidney, and spleen ailments.

The Chinese herbal practitioners use fennel with cinnamon and other herbs to enhance lactation. According to them, fennel increases strength and helps reduce weight. Fennel bulbs are a rich source of energy.

In Ayurveda, fennel is considered good for digestive disorders and as a general tonic. Many of the treatments with fennel in Ayurveda are like those recommended in traditional Chinese medicine.

Fennel water has properties like anise and dill. Mixed with sodium bicarbonate and syrup made with sugar, a gripe water is prepared that provides relief from flatulence in infants. Both the seeds and leaves are used as medicine. Fennel is said to stimulate appetite.

Fennel's medicinal properties have been consolidated to include antioxidative, cytotoxic, anti-inflammatory, anti-microbial, bronchodilatory, estrogenic, diuretic, lithontripic, galactogogue, emmenogogue, anti-thrombotic, hypotensive, gastroprotective, hepatoprotective, memory enhancing, and anti-mutagenic properties (Rahimi et al., 2013).

Fennel seeds were analyzed and were found to be rich in antioxidants with a value of 1.95% (Oktay et al., 2003). Its anti-tumor property has been studied and initial results validate it (Pradhan et al., 2008). The antioxidant and anti-carcinogenic properties were also validated in another study (Mohammad et al., 2011; and de Marino et al., 2007).

The impact of fennel extracts on human leukemia cells was studied and preliminary results were noticed to be positive (Bogucka-Kocka et al., 2008). Another experiment with anethole treatment on Swiss albino mice showed reduction in carcinoma cells (Al-Haribi et al., 1995).

Acetone extracts of fennel seeds were administered in both male and female rats and was observed to cause changes to genital organs (Malini et al., 1985). A study conducted on rats showed fennel seed extracts reduce stress and improve memory (Koppula et al., 2013). Fennel seeds have been shown to have anti-anxiety impact on mice (Kishore et al., 2012).

Fennel extracts given to rabbits tested for their property to reduce eye pressure in glaucoma (Agarwal et al., 2008). The anti-inflammatory, analgesic, and antioxidant activities of fennel seeds were validated (Choi et al., 2004).

The hepatoprotective effect of fennel extracts and its antioxidant properties were studied on wistar rats, and results indicate that the herb is a rich source of antioxidants (Ghanem et al., 2012). The hypolipidemic and anti-atherogenic property of fennel extracts was validated in experiments (Oulmouden et al., 2011).

The dried plant is an insect repellant and helps keeps fleas away. Yellow and brown dyes are obtained from the leaves and flowers too.

Clove – an antioxidant more powerful than blueberry

Clove is a spice that is used both in Chinese and Indian food. It is an ingredient of Chinese five-spice powder and Indian garam masala. It also is an ingredient in the four-spice popular powder used in French cuisine.

The plant is an evergreen tree indigenous to Indonesia, its biggest producer. Other regions that produce cloves are Madagascar, Tanzania, and Sri Lanka. It was only in the 18th century that European colonizers introduced the spice to India. Small areas of clove plantations exist in the country, mostly as a shade crop in the coffee plantations of South India.

The Chinese have been importing cloves for over 2,500 years. Most imports were by sea via the active trade relations between the Maluku Islands of Indonesia and the Southern China sea ports.

There existed an active trade between Indonesia, Sri Lanka, and India from the 3rd millennium BC to the 17th century AD. India was the center of trade during much of this period. Spices and other items were moved from India to Mesopotamia, Egypt, Greece, Rome, and Europe both by sea as well as by land. Arab seamen and traders played an active role in this thriving trade.

The spice trade fell into the hands of the European colonial powers of Holland, Spain, Portugal, France, and finally, the British. Each of these powers established colonies across Africa and Asia. The territories were exploited for spices for sale in Europe.

The North Indonesian Islands were the home of cloves and nutmeg and were converted into near pure spice tree plantations. Large swathes of valuable evergreen forests were destroyed to cultivate these commercial crops.

Cloves grow well in evergreen and semi -evergreen habitats of Southeast Asia, Sri Lanka, South India, and Africa. They thrive in deep, loamy soil rich in humus and in altitudes that are below 1,000 meters from mean sea level. The clove also grows well on laterite soils seen in abundance in the coastal regions of Southern India. The species belongs to the guava family Myrtaceae.

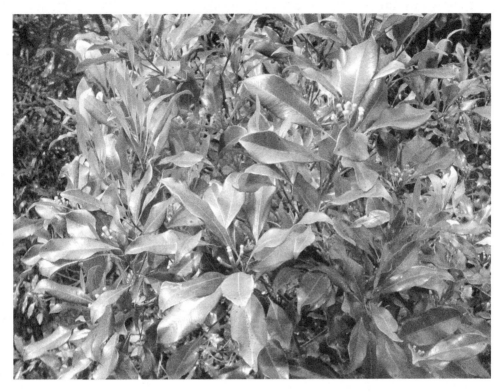

Picture 28 Syzygium aromaticum tree
Photo: Dr Ravikumar, Senior botanist, FRLHT

The tree of Syzygium aromaticum is 8-12 meters tall.

The plants are raised from seed in nurseries before being planted in the field. They start producing fruit and seeds after 15 years of life. The fruits are allowed to ripen and drop down naturally on the soil. They are then soaked in water overnight to soften the outer fruit coat and extract the seed.

It is the aromatic flower buds of the tree that is used as a spice. The flowers are grouped in terminal clusters and harvested just before they open. The buds are picked by hand when they are pink in color. The buds are dried in the sun until they turn brown. They are kept in the shade
at night to protect them from moisture.

The cloves have a hard exterior but are fleshy inside. The essential oil in the buds make for the fleshiness of the clove and is the source of both nutrition and flavor. The spice has a warm, sweet, aromatic, and slightly peppery taste. Even though cloves are cultivated in abundance in the Indonesian islands, their use in local cuisine is limited.

Even though the flowers can be harvested from the seventh year onward, optimal production is reached at years between the fifteenth and twentieth. Yield could easily reach up to 400 kilograms of the spice per hectare of plantation.

Nearly 50% of the clove produced in Indonesia is used in the manufacture of clove cigarettes, quite popular in the region. These cigarettes are exported too.

According to the Food and Agriculture Organization, in 2013, Indonesia produced 98,700 metric tons of cloves, followed by Madagascar with 22,500 MT, Tanzania with 6,950 MT and Sri Lanka with 3,920 MT. China, too, produces a small quantity of cloves. FAO places that at 1,200 MT. The largest producer of Indonesia has been estimated to cultivate cloves over an area of 329,000 hectares.

US imports of clove oil made from leaf, stem, and bark in 2013 has been put at 577.5 metric tons by US International Trade Commission. Of this total quantity, a lion's share of 403 MT came from Indonesia. The Indonesian government estimates put the production of clove oil at 4,800 MT in 2011. The yield from the buds ranges from 11-17%, while that from leaves, stem, and fruit together would average between 4-6%.

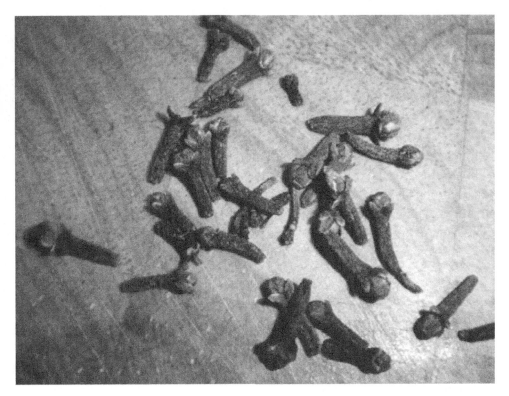

Picture 29 Dried cloves
Photo by: D O'Neil

In Food and Drink

In some parts of Africa, cloves are roasted with coffee for added flavor. In Europe, cloves are used to flavor candy, rice, and meat. It is a popular spice in cuisine of Middle East, South Asia, and Sri Lanka as well as North and East Africa, Mexico, and other Latin American cuisine.

The aroma of the cloves from Zanzibar is said to be the best in the world. During the Han dynasty, courtiers would mask any unpleasant smell from the mouth by chewing cloves. This was a ritual that was practiced when ushered into the presence of the Emperor.

Cloves contain a substantial quantity of eugenol. The eugenol content in clove oil makes up to 70-85%. The ORAC (Oxygen Radical Absorption Capacity) value of cloves has been placed at over 10 million which is 400 times more powerful than the antioxidant contained in blueberry. This high ORAC value makes cloves valuable as both a nutraceutical and in medicine. Cloves are an excellent source of manganese, vitamin K, and dietary fiber.

Cloves can be stored in sealed containers and stay fresh for up to six months. Clove oil is extracted from buds, leaves, stem, fruit, and bark of the plant by distillation. The oil color has a tinge of yellow which turns dark brown as it matures. Cloves are available in trade as whole buds, oil, and a spice powder. The American Herbal Products Association has placed cloves in Class 1 rating which translates to safe for consumption.

In Medicine

Eugenol, the active component, is used across the world by dentists in root canal therapy, temporary fillings, gum pain, and as a mild anesthetic and antibacterial agent. The species is also used in toothpaste, mouthwashes, and chewing gum.

In Chinese traditional medicine, cloves are said to possess a heating property. This is also a belief in India too. Tea infused with cloves, cinnamon, holy basil, and cardamom is drunk for relief when suffering from a cold.

In traditional Chinese medicine, the spice is said to possess anti-fungal, anti-cholera, and anti-diarrheal properties. A poultice made from cloves provides relief in cases of cracked nipples and insect and scorpion bites. Clove helps relieve indigestion.

The spice has an impact on the middle meridian of the body. Its action is on the liver and spleen. In Ayurveda, cloves are recommended as treatment for diabetes, fever, cough, cold, allergy, headache, etc. Clove oil is also used in aromatherapy. It is said to be ant-repellent too.

The clove's medicinal properties and toxicological impacts have been studied. An accidental ingestion of clove essential oil by a seven-month-old infant showed development of central nervous system depression, urinary, and other abnormalities (Lane et al., 1991).

The high ORAC value makes for a high anti-cancer potential. Eugenol, which is the key constituent of clove essential oil, was shown to have anti-cancer property in studies conducted on human leukemia cells (Yoo et al., 2005). The cytotoxic property of eugenol was also demonstrated in experiments conducted on rats (Thomson et al., 1991). The chemo preventive property of the eugenol molecule has also been validated in experiments conducted on albino mice (Kumari et al., 1991).

The anti-inflammatory property of eugenol was validated, with respect to asthma and bronchitis. The anti-inflammatory and vessel relaxation property of the eugenol molecule was studied and validated in experiments on rats (Damiani et al., 2003). The anti-inflammatory and chemo preventive property of eugenol has also been demonstrated in an experiment conducted by Kim et al. in 2003.

The action of 30 traditional herbs used in Chinese medicine for their antibacterial actions was studied against six Helicobacter pylori strains. H. pylori is said to cause ulcers and severe gastritis. Clove essential oil was found to have a pronounced anti-H. pylori action (Li et al., 2005). A significant reduction of food poisoning causing enterotoxins produced by Staphylococcus aureus bacteria was observed in a study conducted in 2004 (Smith-Palmer et al., 2004).

Anti-fungal activity due to the presence of eugenol and thymol was observed in experiments conducted on yeast cells (Bennis et al., 2004). Other experiments demonstrated the anti-candidal activity of eugenol (Chami et al., 2005). Candida is a yeast that causes vaginal infection. Experiments in rats have supported the anti-candidal properties of eugenol (Chami et al., 2004).

Anti-microbial effects of clove were observed in experiments conducted on soft cheese and other food (Leuschner et al., 2003). The anti-fungal properties of spice essential oils that included cloves has been demonstrated in experiments conducted on bakery products (Guynot et al., 2003). The antibacterial property of molecules in cloves has been further demonstrated in experiments conducted on apple juice (Friedman et al., 2004).

Molecules in cloves were found to possess properties that can control hypertension, reduce cholesterol levels, and in general be helpful in cardiovascular diseases (Somova et al., 2003). However, human consumption of naturally existing methyleugenol has properties like the known carcinogen safrole. In experiments on rats, the molecule was seen to eliminate rapidly from the human system in trials conducted in the US raising questions about the safety of clove essential oil for human use. But conclusive evidence to this effect is still lacking (Schecter et al., 2004).

The insecticidal property of clove oil was demonstrated in experiments (Choi et al., 2003). The oil was observed to be effective in checking growth of head lice, Pediculus capititis (Yang et al., 2003).

The local anesthesial property of clove essential oil has been demonstrated in experiments (Alqareer et al., 2006). The anesthetic effect was comparable to benzocaine, a chemical already in use. The anti-allergic and anti-pyretic (fever reduction) properties have been proven too. The action of the molecule was found to be like the anti-pyretic chemical acetaminophen (Feng et al. 1987).

Sudhir Ahluwalia

CHAPTER VI

MARIJUANA – Fiber, intoxicant and medicine

The hemp plant—Cannabis sativa—leaves, flowers, stem, and seed are more in the news for its use as an intoxicating and hallucinating product than its major use as a source of fiber and oil. The species has multiple cultivars and varieties each with differing properties that determine the end use of the plant.

History

Hemp is one of the earliest agricultural crops known to man (Sagan, 1977). Pottery discovered from an ancient village site c. 7000 BC in Taiwan revealed its use to make hemp cord. Hemp fiber wrapped around a baby skeleton was discovered at Catahoyuk in Turkey c. 9000 BC.[30]

Cannabis seed and oil were probably used as food in China since at least 6000 BC. The earliest use of hemp in medicine goes back to the time of the Chinese emperor Sheng Nung c. 2727 BC. It was said to be popular as it possesses both yin and yang properties (Deitch, 2003). Excavations in the Yanghai tombs in the Xinjiang-Uighur Autonomous Region of China have uncovered a 2700-year-old grave in which cannabis was found. The cannabis was probably used as medicine or for its psychoactive properties (Russo, 2008).

There are references to marijuana in the Chinese pharmacopeia that go back to 1500 BC (National Institute of Drug Abuse – Marijuana Research Findings – 1976, 1977). The Chinese were said to use cannabis to treat diarrhea, dysentery, and to stimulate appetite.

The use of cannabis in India probably goes back to the Vedic times (c.

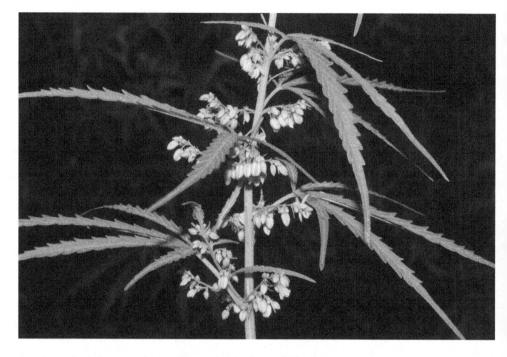

Picture 30 Cannabis plant
Photo by: Dr Ravikumar Sr Botanist FRLHT

1800 BC onwards), as mentioned in the Atharvaveda.

The Zendavesta, which is the Holy Book of the Zorastrians (composed around 700-600 BC), has numerous references to bhang (local Indian name for recreational marijuana). It is referred to therein as the good narcotic. Sushrutasamhita mentions use of cannabis as an anti-phlegmatic and as a cure for leprosy.

Pliny the Elder refers to the use of the plant both for rope-making and as an analgesic (23-79 AD). Dioscorides lists it as a medicine (c. 70 AD).

While there are some scholars who believe that cannabis was an ingredient in the Holy Anointing Oils used by the ancient Jews c. 1450 BC, my analysis of the plants and spices used in the Anointing Oil does not support this conclusion (Holy Herbs, Sudhir Ahluwalia, 2017).

Ancient Jews used cannabis both as an intoxicant and in medicine. It was a popular medicinal plant in Pharaonic Egypt too. Pollen of cannabis was discovered in the nostrils of mummy of Ramesses II. The plant was said to be used by Ancient Egyptians to treat glaucoma, for cooling the uterus, and as an enema.

There are repeated references to the use of cannabis as a source of fiber, in paper-making, textile, as an intoxicant, and medicine all throughout history. Queen Victoria is said to have used cannabis to relieve severe pain that she suffered from menstrual cramps.

Marijuana was said to have been first brought into the US by the Jamestown settlers in 1611. George Washington and Thomas Jefferson are said to have cultivated hemp for medicine and for recreational smoking. Marijuana was added to the US Pharmacopeia in 1850 where it is listed as treatment for neuralgia, tetanus, leprosy, dysentery, uterine bleeding, and many other ailments. Most hemp imported into the country came from India and Madagascar.

Many US states, starting with Massachusetts in 1911, progressively prohibited the use of cannabis. Many other European countries like the UK, too prohibited and criminalized its use.

The American Medical Association opposed the promulgation of the Marihuana Tax Act in 1937 and supported research on medical cannabis. In 1961, the UN Convention recommended prohibition of use of cannabis.

While the movement to ban use of cannabis in the US and Europe continued on the one hand, on the other, the National Institute of Drug Abuse (NIDA) contracted University of Mississippi to grow cannabis to meet demands of research. Research Triangle Institute was contracted to manufacture and distribute cannabis cigarettes for use to provide relief to individuals suffering from excessive pain.

There continued a prolonged and continuous battle between supporters and opponents of the use of marijuana for medical purposes in various law courts of the US, Canada, and Europe. Over time, the proponents for use of marijuana for medical purposes have won the fight against the ban lobbyists. Today, many states in the US have permitted growing and use of marijuana for medical and research purposes. In some countries like the Netherlands, recreational use of marijuana too is permitted.

To distinguish industrial hemp from recreational cannabis, the US Congress re-introduced the Industrial Hemp Farming Act of 2015 which would exclude industrial hemp from being regulated as a controlled substance. Countries like China and Russia, on the other hand have never proscribed cultivation of cannabis for either industrial or other use.

Botany

Cannabis sativa and Cannabis indica are sources of industrial hemp and medicinal marijuana, respectively. Cannabis belongs to the Urticaceae family. There are large numbers of cultivars of Cannabis, many of which are named after the locality in which they are found.

Cannabis sativa is also used in medicine and as a recreational weed. The variety used for medical and recreational purposes are tall and thin with narrower leaves and a light green color. Hemp plants from Europe are short with broader and greener leaves and no psychoactive properties.

Marijuana-yielding plants are morphologically nearly indistinguishable from industrial hemp cultivars, but marijuana varieties are more branched and bushy whereas industrial hemp producing plants are straight with fewer branches.

Cannabis plants are annual herbs. Plant height rarely goes beyond five meters.

Leaves are palmate with lanceolate, serrate leaflets 10 centimeters long and 1.5 centimeter broad. The species is probably native to the Central Asian region. It is cultivated across many parts of Asia, Europe, and China. It is an introduced species in the US and North Africa.

Cannabis plants can be seen growing in the wild in degraded forest sites in India. Cannabis plants can be seen growing in the wild along roads and can survive in a wide range of soil and climate conditions. The resistance of the species to ground frost and waterlogging is quite low.

The plant is propagated mainly by seed. Sowing is done in early spring. It is a vigorously growing species that rapidly crowds out weeds, needing only a little care. Rarely does one need to irrigate the hemp crop.

Interbreeding is easy and common in nature. Most natural crops are composed of multiple cultivars, each with its own set of characteristics. Cultivars good for fiber have longer stalks, branch very little, and yield only small quantities of seed. Profusely seeding varieties are short and mature early. Drug-yielding varieties too are short. They are much branched and have smaller, dark-green leaves.

As the plant is a rapid interbreeder, industrial hemp, oilseeds, and medicinal or recreational marijuana yielding plants should be cultivated in separate plots. Cross-pollination affects the content of THC (tetrahydrocannibol), the primary psychoactive molecule in the plant. Higher levels of THC will make the crop unsuitable for industrial hemp production.

Cultivation of varieties with high THC content is strictly controlled in Europe and North America. However, there are no such restrictions placed in Asia.

Industrial Hemp

Hemp fiber is obtained from the bast of Cannabis sativa. The fiber is a good conductor of heat. It is also known to possess natural antibacterial properties.

The THC content in fiber yielding cultivars is under 1%, optimally under 0.3%. Best fiber yield ranges between 15-25%. The fiber is used in textile, rope, and paper making.

The earliest paper was made in China from hemp fiber. This fiber is biodegradable and used to manufacture biodegradable plastic: hemp plastic. Hemp fiber is fine and soft with cotton-like properties. Hemp when blended with human-made fibers is called hemp viscose. Hemp rayon staple is ideal for cotton textiles. Hemp industrial and hemp viscose fiber when mixed in the ratio of 3:1 makes it suitable for use in cotton textiles.

China is the largest producer of industrial hemp, producing nearly 80% of the total global production. The Hemp Industries Association puts the worldwide annual production of hemp at around 55,700 metric tons. The second major producer of hemp after China is France accounting for 14% of the world production. No industrial hemp is produced in the US.

There are 30 hemp producing countries.

Crop density affects yield and fiber content. Yield varies from 2.5 to 14 metric tons of dry retted stalks per hectare. During the retting process, fiber is separated from the other organic matter. The process takes from 14 to 28 days. The cooler the weather, the longer it takes to ret. Most retting is done in the open.

Fiber is present on the outer rind of the stalk and must be separated from the inner woody part. For this, the stalks need to be dry after which the woody parts are split into short pieces. These, called hurds, are passed through multiple rollers to separate the fiber from the wood.

Hemp is cultivated mainly for its fiber and oilseed. The fiber is used in fabric making. The seed is used in food. The value of the global hemp industry is estimated at $1.5 trillion. Hemp Industries Association puts the total retail value of hemp products in use in the US in 2012 to over $500 million. About $156-171 million of this was used in hemp food and body care products.

Paper made from hemp lasts five times longer than paper made from wood. Pre-1900 books were printed largely on hemp paper. The first two drafts of the Declaration of Independence of the US were written on paper made from hemp.

Hemp Seed and Oil

Hemp oil is extracted from seeds and is almost free of THC. Hemp seeds have a hard-outer shell and a soft inner kernel. Oil is extracted by pressing the seed or the whole hemp plant. Hemp seeds are made of 30-35% oil by weight. There are some varieties where oil percent can be as high as 50%.

Hemp seed is rich in protein with all the 20 amino acids essential for the human body. The oil is rich in omega acids. Hemp seeds have a short life due to the presence of unsaturated fat; they must be refrigerated and stored away from light and heat.

Milk from hemp is a dairy-free alternative of high nutrition value. Several products are made from hemp seed by blending these with milk, milk-based products, oils, grain flour, etc. They are blended into baked products like cakes, made into granola bars, etc. Hemp butter is used as a spread.

Seeds have a nutty taste like flaxseed and can be eaten raw or mixed in bread.

Hemp seed and oil is used in the manufacture of moisturizers and lotions. They are blended with other oils and cream to make soap. The oil hydrates the skin and nourishes it by increasing circulation. Unrefined oil has a green tinge and nutty flavor. The shelf life of the oil can be enhanced after refining. Refined hemp oil is colorless.

The oil can be used as biodiesel though that is not yet being done on an industrial scale. It is also used in manufacture of low emission paints. Petroleum-based paint products decompose over time, emitting harmful chemicals, and hemp-based paints are preferred as they are more eco-and health-friendly.

185

Medical or Recreational Marijuana

It is Cannabis Indica that is cultivated for use as marijuana. Cannabis Indicahas its origin in the Hindu Kush mountain range region of South Asia. Much of this cultivation is done in Afghanistan, Tibet, and nearby areas. The whole plant from flowers, seed, shoots, and leaves are used as marijuana.

Jean Baptiste Lamarck, in 1785, identified Cannabis Indica from hemp plants found growing in Northern India. It has a resinous body that protects it from the harsh winters of the region. The plants have higher intoxicating properties. Locals make hashish from this species. Marijuana's therapeutic properties were recognized in Western medicine only in 1800s.

Recreational Use

In South Asia, leaves of marijuana plants are hand-picked and squeezed to make small balls which is locally called bhang. This is sold during Holi (spring festival celebrated in North and West India) in February or March every year. Bhang, mixed in milk or yoghurt, makes for a potent psychedelic drink.

When crushed, a resin exudes from leaves and small twigs, which, in dried form is called charas. A narcotic combination made from resin, the flowering portion and foliage, is called ganja and hashish. The flowers of the female plant contain the maximum toxicity. Continuous selection has led to development of cultivars with more potent narcotic property. Hashish is the more concentrated and potent form and is made into balls, cakes, or sticks.

Hashish and charas are both smoked. These are popular with marijuana lovers and addicts. In India, there is a religious association to hashish and ganja smoking as followers of the Hindu God Shiva, who is believed to have enjoyed marijuana, are often seen smoking hash during the religious festival of Kumbh celebrated on the banks of the river Ganges once every twelve years.

The refined oily extract of the cannabis plant is called hash oil. The THC content of hash oil averages around 15%. The oil is amber to dark brown in color and smoked in combination with tobacco or marijuana.

THC (delta-9-tetrahydrocanninol) is the mind-altering chemical in marijuana. Dr. Raphael Mechoulam, Professor of Medicinal Chemistry at the Hebrew University of Jerusalem, is said to have first identified THC as the main psychoactive component of cannabis in 1964. He also was the first to synthesize THC.

According to NORML (US National Organization for the Reform of Marijuana Laws), marijuana is the third most popular recreational drug in use in America after alcohol and tobacco.

Institutions like NORML in the US lobby to permit recreational and medical use of marijuana. There are several studies, which, on the other hand, have repeatedly shown that marijuana is injurious to human health. In a testimony to a US Congress subcommittee, Nora D. Volkow, MD, on June 24, 2014, stated that "scientific research has shown significant adverse effects (of marijuana) on health and well-being of people."

According to the 2013 Monitoring the Future survey of high school students, marijuana usage was found to be highest among high school students in the US. There is a growing perception among young people that marijuana is a relatively harmless drug. Even though, marijuana plants are grown in Sou th Asia, they do not evoke the same amount of interest as they do in the US and Europe. The popularity of marijuana usage is very limited in South Asia. THC content which is the marijuana's main psychoactive ingredient has been rising. The potency of an average marijuana cigarette has increased from 3% THC in 1990s to 12.5% in 2013. Hash oil with over 80% THC content has been produced. Average content of THC in the hash oil found in the US is now over 50%. Intoxication from marijuana is raising the risk of automobile accidents (Volkow, 2014).

Medicinal Use

The synthetic form of THC going under the trade name of Marinol was approved for medical use in May 1985 and was used to treat nausea and vomiting caused by chemotherapy. This product was approved by US FDA to treat anorexia in patients with AIDS too (Eddy, 2010).

Marijuana has both short- and long-term effects on the brain. The THC in marijuana, when smoked or ingested in drink and food, is known to pass into the bloodstream quickly. The intoxication lasts for 30 minutes to one hour after ingestion.

The drug activates the brain, and there is a feeling of a high, change in mood, impaired body movement, impaired memory, and difficulty with thinking and problem solving. Long-term effects can permanently impact the human brain.

Marijuana smoke irritates the lungs and impairs breathing. Heart rate is faster and stays up for three hours after use. In those susceptible to heart ailments, this can trigger heart attacks. The drug can impact the development of the brain of a fetus and should be avoided by pregnant women.

Marijuana use can lead to hallucinations, paranoia, schizophrenia, depression, and anxiety, and marijuana tends to addictive (Anthony, 1994; Lopez-Quintero, 2011).

According to the Indian Central Science and Industrial Research publication, Cannabis plants are used as tonic, intoxicant, stomachic, anti-spasmodic, analgesic, narcotic, sedative, and anodyne in folk medicine. Seeds and leaves are used to treat cancerous ulcers and tumors.

A decoction of the root is said to help remedy hard tumors and knots in the joints. Other folk uses include treating delirium, depression,diarrhea, dysentery, dysmenorrhea, epilepsy, fever, gonorrhea, migraine, neuralgia, rheumatism toothache, uteral prolapse, etc.

Cannabinoids found in marijuana were studied for their antioxidant and neuroprotectant property. A US Department of Health and Human Services patent US 6630507 B1 was awarded to Aidan J. Hampson, Julius Axelrod, and Maurizio Grimaldi in October 2003. The abstract citation is reproduced below:

Cannabinoids have been found to have antioxidant properties, unrelated to NMDA (N-methyl-D-aspartate) receptor antagonism. This new-found property makes cannabinoids useful in the treatment and prophylaxis of wide variety of oxidation associated diseases, such as ischemic, age-related, inflammatory and autoimmune diseases. The cannabinoids are found to have application as neuroprotectants, for example in limiting neurological damage following ischemic insults, such as stroke and trauma, or in the treatment of neurodegenerative diseases, such as Alzheimer's disease, Parkinson's disease and HIV dementia. Nonpsychoactive cannabinoids, such as cannabidiol, are particularly advantageous to use because they avoid toxicity that is encountered with psychoactive cannabinoids at high doses useful in the method of the present invention...

Hemp resin has a molecule combination called cannabinone which is soluble in alcohol and ether. Cannabinol separated from the resin is a volatile alkaloid-resembling nicotine. Cannabis contains choline, eugenol, guaiacol, nicotine, and piperidine, all listed as toxins by the National Institute of Occupational Safety and Health (C.S.I.R., 1948-1976).

The association between marijuana use and adverse cardiac events like myocardial infarction, sudden cardiac death, cardiomyopathy, stroke, transient ischemic attack and cannabis arteritis has been made (Thomas et al., 2014). The association between marijuana and polysubstance abusers and higher prospects of HIV infections was made in a study conducted in the US (Andrade et al., 2013).

The long-term effects of cannabis use on cognitive functions have also been studied and established (Crean et al., 2011). Lynsky (2000) has studied the effects of adolescent cannabis use on educational attainment and noted a negative correlation. Further, the relationship between marijuana initiation and dropping out from school has been established (Bray et al., 2000).

Researchers have consistently observed that cannabis use is associated with the inset of schizophrenia later in life. Some individuals are observed to be more vulnerable to schizophrenia when compared to others. Studies on animals have indicated that use during adolescence carries high risk (Casadio et al., 2011).

Exposure of the fetus to marijuana impacts the development of its brain.

A study conducted by Tashkin (2013) could not associate respiratory impairment with even prolonged smoking of marijuana. Probable association with higher levels of THC may still exist.

There does appear to be consensus on the psychological impact of marijuana, as with any drug that has psychoactive components and action. Components of marijuana are under investigation about its effect as a treatment for autoimmune diseases and malignancy (Owen et al., 2014).

The association of marijuana with lung and upper-aerodigestive track cancers could not be established in a California-based case control study (Hashibe et al., 2006). However, another case control study, also conducted in California, has shown an association between marijuana use and nonseminonma and mixed tumors (Lacson et al., 2012).

CHAPTER VII

GINSENG
(research supported medicinal properties)

Ginseng has been in use in Chinese medicine for millennia. Ginseng comes from the fleshy roots of perennial slow-growing plants belonging to 11 different species and two different genera. There are three popular varieties—Asian, American, and Siberian.

Asian or Korean ginseng is the oldest. The most famous and commonly found of the ginseng comes from Panax ginseng. American ginseng comes from Panax quinquefolius. Siberian ginseng is from a different genus: Eleutherococcus senticosus.

Three more species of the Panax genus are used in traditional medicine: Panax vietnamensis (Vietnamese Ginseng), Panax japonicas (Japanese ginseng), and Panax notoginseng (Pseudoginseng). Both Panax and Eleutherococcus species belong to the Araliaceae family.

Outside of this family, but still called ginseng, are the Malaysian ginseng (Eurycoma longifolia), Peruvian ginseng (Lepidium meyenii), Southern ginseng (Gynostemma pentaphyllum), Brazilian ginseng (Pfaffia paniculata), Kerala ginseng (Trichopus zeylanicus), Thai ginseng (Kaempferia parviflora), Nam ginseng (Dracena angustifolia), and Ashwangandha or Indian ginseng (Withania somnifera). A cheap substitute for Panax ginseng comes from Codonopsis pilosula.

There are 3,944 prescriptions having ginseng as an ingredient in the Korean Clinical Pharmacopeia that has been in place since 1610 AD. Ginseng's name comes from the Chinese word renshen translated as "man root."

History

Panax ginseng is cultivated in the Manchurian mountain region of China where it was discovered over 5,000 years ago. Probably, ginseng was used as food until it became known for its strength-giving and rejuvenating properties also.

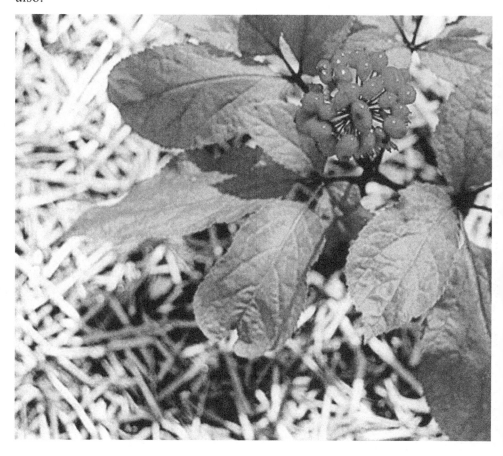

Picture 31 Panax ginseng plant in fruit
Photo by: By FloraFarm GmbH / Katharina Lohrie

The benefits of ginseng were first documented at the time of the Liang Dynasty (220-589 AD). Ginseng is an ingredient in an entire spectrum of traditional Chinese medicine herbal medicines. It is also used in soaps, lotions, and creams.

The herb was popular with Chinese emperors, who paid for it in gold. Overexploitation led to the near disappearance of the plant. On the back of this, an ancient trade in ginseng with Korea began from the 3rd century AD. The Silk Road was a popular route for this trade between China and the rest of the trading world.

In America, Native American tribes like the Iroquois, Menomonee, Cherokee, and the Creeks all valued the herb for its curative powers, but cultivation of ginseng in the US began in 20th century only. Widespread cultivation has helped save the species from imminent extinction.

Trade and Production

The four largest producers of ginseng are China, South Korea, Canada, and the US. These together make for 99% of global production or 80,080 metric tons. (Baeg et al., 2013). The Chinese production is 44,749 metric tons, South Korea produced 27,480 tons, Canada produced 6,486 tons, and the US 1,054 tons (Korea Ministry for Food, Agriculture, Forestry and Fisheries, Ginseng statistic data, 2010).

China is the largest producer of ginseng. Both China and Korea are also the largest consumers of the herb. The primary use in these countries is as a nutrition supplement. Korea and Canada both export extensively to the US too. Ginseng is said to be consumed in 35 countries around the world (Baeg et al., 2013).

American ginseng is indigenous to North America. It is found growing across deciduous forest regions of Eastern US. Farmers started cultivating the herb in the 1970s. Marathon County in Wisconsin produces over 90% of ginseng grown in the country. It is also widely grown in the Ontario province of Canada. Collection of the root from the wild is permitted in the US once the plant attains five years of age or more.

Cultivation of ginseng is done by dibbling the seed in the ground. The plant, in four to five years, grows to a height of one to two feet. The rhizome, which is the commercial part of the plant, develops in –four to five years. In the first three years, the roots reach a size of three to eight inches and a weight of one ounce.

Trade in ginseng is regulated in the US and standards for harvesting and export set. Ginseng is accorded a Generally Recognized as Safe (GRAS) status by the US FDA.

It is the root of ginseng that is used in traditional medicine. The root is tuberous and has a sweetish taste that leaves a bitter aftertaste. The herb has a light-colored, fork-shaped root. The stalk is long with oval-shaped leaves. The plant produces greenish, yellow flowers and pea-sized, crimson berry fruits.

Ginseng is of two types. One type, white ginseng, is dried and untreated rhizome. When fresh, it has a whitish color which turns brown on drying. Red ginseng is the processed plant. The roots are preserved by exposing them to steam, and the heat leads to change in color to red. Red ginseng can withstand heat.

Older roots are used in preparing red ginseng, which is considered more potent than white ginseng. Both Panax and American ginseng can be heat-treated to produce red ginseng. In addition to fresh, white, and red ginseng, another variety consumed in Korea is Taekuksam which is fresh rhizome blanched in water and then dried.

The active ingredient ginsenosides is common to the ginseng of the Panax genus. Ginsenosides are a group of steroidal saponins and over 100 ginsenosides have been identified which have similar molecular structures and are bioactive compounds. The quantity of ginsenosides starts decreasing after the plant is older than five years of age. The ideal time of harvest of ginseng is put between four to six years. Today, ginseng is used largely in medicine.

Younger ginseng plants are used in food. Ginseng is used to flavor beverages, toothpaste, chewing gum, and cigarettes. It is estimated that over six million Americans use ginseng.[31] The herb is sold as crystals, extracts, in capsules, and as the whole root. The product is marketed in Asian and health food stores in the US.

Medicinal Use

In Asia, in particular, China and Korea, ginseng is believed to possess miraculous restorative and strength-enhancing properties. In the US, the FDA has not recognized it as medicine, but it is accepted it a GRAS (Generally Recognized as Safe) nutraceutical.

Traditionally, ginseng is regarded as both a physical and mental restorant. It is said to improve the cognitive ability of patients, improve the quality of life and behavior. Ginsenoides and other constituents in ginseng possess immunosuppressive properties. It is also said to be an aphrodisiac. Other medicinal properties include ability to improve concentration, memory, physical efficiency, and athletic endurance.

In Western medicine, Panax ginseng is simulative while in traditional Chinese medicine, it is used to induce a feeling of calm. It is also used to treat ailments related to heart and blood vessels, diabetes, etc. Studies conducted on healthy individuals given Panax ginseng doses of 200 mg of extract daily showed increased QTc interval[32] and decreased diastolic blood pressure two hours after ingestion on the first day of therapy (Caron et al., 2002).

---

31   https://www.drugs.com/npp/ginseng.html
32   The heart's electrical currents are measured by the interval of Q and T electrical waves.
The faster the heart rate, the closer is the interval between these waves.

Cognitive enhancement ability tests with herbal treatment with Panax ginseng were conducted on healthy volunteers who had fasted overnight. The results confirm that the herb possesses glucoregulatory and cognitive performance-enhancing properties (Scholey et al., 2016).

It has also been shown that a dose-dependent improvement in memory quality was seen in experiments conducted on volunteers who were administered Ginkgo biloba and Panax ginseng treatment. The highest improvement was observed in those who were given the highest dose (Kennedy et al., 2001). Positive results were also observed when Ginkgo biloba and Panax ginseng were given to the volunteer patients with neurasthenic complaints (Wesnes et al., 1997).

On the other hand, no memory or cognitive improvement was noticed in post-menopausal women volunteers. In the study, volunteers were administered a combination of Ginkgo biloba and Panax ginseng called gincosan over a sustained period (Hartley et al., 2013).

Panax ginseng is often sold in combination with guarana (Paullinia cupana) which has high levels of caffeine. A combination of the two herbs was given to the subjects of a study. The results showed increased speed of memory task performance. However, there was little evidence of modulated memory increase (Kennedy et al., 2004).

Lee et al. (2003) observed that red ginseng leads to improvement of cognitive functions in patients suffering from Alzheimer's disease. An open label clinical trial showed ginseng helped improve cognitive functions in such cases. Ginseng was being administered as an adjuvant[33] (Heo et al., 2008).

Traditionally, treatment with Panax ginseng has been used to lower blood glucose levels and improve cognitive abilities. A double-blind, placebo-controlled trial confirms that Panax ginseng may possess glucoregulatory properties and can enhance cognitive performance (Reay et al., 2005).

---

33   Applied after initial treatment for cancer, especially to suppress secondary tumour formation.

Another study by the same group of scientists showed that single doses of Panax ginseng reduce blood glucose levels and improve cognitive performance during sustained mental activity (Reay et al., 2006).

A clinical trial with patients of the age range 60-61 years and age-related memory impairment cases was conducted. This group was administered ginseng containing vitamin supplements, and the results indicated improvement of cognitive ability (Neri et al., 1995).

On the other hand, when the subjective mood and aspects of working memory processes in healthy volunteers were studied following treatment with Panax ginseng, no change was observed (Reay et al., 2010).

Another study indicated that mental health and social functioning of patients improved after four weeks of therapy with Panax ginseng. This improvement attenuated with continued use (Ellis et al., 2002). Similar dose-dependant action of combination therapy with Ginkgo biloba and Panax ginseng was observed in healthy young volunteers (Scholey et al., 2002).

A study was conducted on healthy elderly individuals who are more likely to consume herbal supplements. It was observed that patients administered with Panax ginseng showed higher prospects of ability of the body to break down toxic chemicals in the body (Gurley et al., 2005).

The use of ginseng as an aphrodisiac was validated in a study conducted on women volunteers who were keen to improve their sexual desire. The results were compared with a control group who were on a placebo. Notable improvement in sexual desire, reduction of vaginal dryness, frequency of sexual intercourse and orgasm, and clitoral sensation was noted (Ito et al., 2001). No side effects were observed in the individuals.

ArginMax is a combination containing L-arginine, ginseng, ginkgo, dimiana, multivitamins, and minerals. A double-blind, placebo-controlled study to determine the role of dietary supplementation on sexual function in women of differing menopausal status was conducted. The results indicate that this combination could be an alternative to hormone therapy during menopause (Ito et al., 2006). Another study showed that red ginseng extracts may be used as an alternative medicine in menopausal women to improve their sexual life. (Oh et al., 2010).

Ginseng's ability to help alleviate erectile dysfunction was validated (Kim et al., 2009). But, a systematic review with red ginseng for treating erectile dysfunctionality presented uncertain results (Jan et al., 2008). Korean red ginseng was observed to be an effective alternative remedy for treating male erectile dysfunction (Hong et al., 2002).

Ginseng is traditionally not recommended for pregnant women. A trial conducted on mice showed defects on the embryo when given ginseng. It is, therefore, recommended that women should not take ginseng in the first three months of pregnancy (Liu et al., 2005).

Ginseng should not be taken without medical advice. The herb has side-effects and can cause headaches, nausea, restlessness, elevated heart rate, sleeplessness, irritability, blurred vision, edema, diarrhea, excessive menopausal bleeding, etc.

Ginseng has been shown to react negatively to certain drugs. Studies conducted on a group of patients who have undergone cardiac-valve replacement and taking warfarin, the anti-coagulant drug, showed adverse interaction with red ginseng. Ginseng supplements should be taken under medical supervision so that adverse reactions with other drugs can be prevented (Lee et al., 2010).

Han et al. (1998) observed that red ginseng could be an adjuvant to treating hypertension. A study on 45 cardiac patients suggested that red ginseng and digoxin had a synergistic effect for treating congestive heart failure. Red ginseng was found to be an effective and safe adjuvant without any side effects (Ding et al., 1995).

Ginsenosides present in ginseng were shown to cause adverse interactions with multiple drugs (Hao et al., 2010). Individuals who were given Panax ginseng and administered midazolam and fexofenadine allopathic medicine showed an adverse impact on the liver (Malati et al., 2012).

Similarly, herbal supplements from ginseng including Siberian ginseng and Ashwagandha (Indian ginseng) showed adverse interactions with the cardiac-stimulant digoxin (Dasgupta et al., 2008). Prolonged use of ginseng and related products was observed to cause menometrorrhagia (hormone imbalance related uterine changes that lead to excessive menstrual bleeding) and tachycardia (enhanced heart beat). Withdrawal of the consumption stopped these adverse reactions in this patient (Kabalak et al., 2004).

Panax ginseng is often dispensed as a complementary remedy to patients receiving anti-retroviral drugs but resulted in acute elevation of liver enzymes and marked jaundice. A study on such patients revealed that withdrawal of ginseng lozenges led to progressive improvement and reduction of liver damage (Mateo-Carrasco et al., 2012).

Ginseng has been traditionally considered to improve strength and stamina. The findings of the study investigating this does not support the claim as ginseng failed to improve physical performance and heart-rate recovery of individuals undergoing repeated bouts of exhausting exercise (Engels et al., 2003; and Kalputana et al., 2007). Another double-blind, placebo-controlled study on people suffering from functional fatigue was conducted with Pharmaton capsules (these capsules have ginseng as a main ingredient). This study's results indicate that symptoms of functional fatigue were alleviated (LeGal et al., 1996).

However, clinical studies conducted on a cohort of menopausal women did indicate that some quality of life parameters did show beneficial changes from use of ginseng. The parameters would include overall health, physical and psychological well-being etc. Other physiological parameters did not show much change. The authors of the study recommended further study to validate these findings (Wiklund et al., 1999).

Red ginseng is traditionally also believed to have antioxidant, immunostimulatory, and anti-aging properties. A red ginseng extract was applied on female volunteers to see if facial wrinkles on the skin can reduced with positive results (Cho et al., 2009).

Ginseng is claimed to be effective in controlling type-2 diabetes conditions (Ni et al., 2010), improves quality of life in cancer patients (Kim et al., 2006), and improves lipid profile (Shin et al., 2011). A Korean study claims that ginseng use could have hypolipidemic potential (Kim et al., 2003). Most papers supporting these claims have been made in Korean and Chinese language studies. Studies conducted by researchers outside of the region and published in other languages did not adequately support these findings (Kim et al., 2011).

Oral ginseng therapy was observed to not improve Beta-cell function in obese patients with diabetes (Reeds et al., 2011). A three-gram dosage of American ginseng was observed to reduce postprandial glycemia in type-2 diabetic patients. This indicates the possibility of use of this herb in controlling diabetes (Vuksan et al., 2000).

It was observed in a clinical trial that prolonged administration of powdered red ginseng extract for three-years and more exerted significant effect on preventing the incidence of non-organ specific human cancers in males (Yun et al., 2010). Ginseng was used as a complementary therapy in breast cancer patients. A cohort of 1,455 breast cancer patients was studied from the Shanghai Breast Cancer institution and results indicate that ginseng use after cancer was diagnosed showed positive association with the quality of life of these patients (Cui et al., 2006).

Ginsenoside Rb1 is a molecule present in ginseng. Studies conducted by Lee et al. (2003) showed that it acts as a weak phytoestrogen in patients having breast cancer cells, a property that could help alleviate cancer conditions. The impact of ginseng on the chemo preventive action of antioxidants in smokers indicated that the use of the herb can help reduce the risk of cancer and other diseases caused by free radicals associated with smoking (Lee et al., 1998).

Panax ginseng when heat-treated yields a mixture of saponins with potent antioxidative properties. This neo-gensing, as it is called, when administered to induced-tumors in rats showed inhibition of skin tumors (Keum et al., 2000).

To understand if Korean red ginseng is beneficial to patients undergoing HIV anti-retroviral therapy (Sung et al., 2009) conducted a study on such patients. This study supports the theory that the product has a beneficial effect.

A protein isolated from the roots of Chinese ginseng was studied for its action against fungi like Coprinus comatus and Fusarium oxysporum. The study also indicated inhibitory activity against human immunodeficiency virus. Its anti-fungal property was also noted in all cases except against Rhizoctonia solani(Ng et al., 2001).

Lee et al. (2009) study observed that red ginseng could be used to reduce bad breath post-eradication of Helicobacter pylori stomach infection. H. pyloriinfections cause gastric ulcers and severe acidity. After the eradication of the infection, bad breath (halitosis) was observed in patients.

Traditionally, it has been believed in Korean and Chinese herbal medicine that ginseng helps against respiratory ailments. A systematic review of studies, both in English and Chinese, was conducted to study the impact of the herb on chronic obstructive pulmonary disease and the results show evidence of improvement of lung functions and quality of life (An et al., 2011). Ginseng could be a possible natural medicine which, in conjunction with other forms of treatment, will help against cystic fibrosis and Pseudomonas aeruginosa lung infection patients (Pseudomonas aeruginosa bacteria causes pneumonia) (Song et al., 1998).

Ginseng was seen to reduce prostaglandin E2 levels (Kase et al., 1998) and stimulates pituitary-adrenocortical system, affecting the hormonal system of the body (Hiai et al., 1979). A study conducted by Ryu et al. (1995) showed that consumption of ginseng in large quantities led to the development of cerebral arteritis in women. An association of use of a ginseng-based face cream and menopausal bleeding was observed by Hopkins et al. (1998).

Many of the properties indicated in scientific studies conducted in Korea and China would be best revalidated in other parts of the world before any definitive conclusion on the miraculous medicinal properties of ginseng is fully accepted.

BIBLIOGRAPHY

INTRODUCTION

Sudhir Ahluwalia – Nutrigenomics – The next generation nutraceuticals -http://www.naturalproductsinsider.com/blogs/ supplement-perspectives/2016/09/nutrigenomics-the-next-generation-nutraceuticals.aspx

Sudhir Ahluwalia – 3 D Bioprinted Human Tissue Applications for Natural Products Industry - http://www.naturalproductsinsider.com/articles/2016/10/3-d-bioprinted-human-tissue-applications-for-natu. aspx

Sudhir Ahluwalia – The Global Nutraceuticals Market – Case study from Canada – http://www.naturalproductsinsider.com/ articles/2016/05/the-global-nutraceutical-market-case-study-from-c. aspx

CHAPTER 1 HISTORY OF HERBS AND HERBAL TRADE

Saul, H., Madella, M., Fischer, A., Glykou, A., Hartz, S., & Craig, O. E. (2013). Phytoliths in pottery reveal the use of spice in European prehistoric cuisine. PloS one, 8(8), e70583.

Arunima Kashyap & Steve Weber. 2010. Harappan plant use revealed by starch grains from Farmana, India. Antiquity Project Gallery 84(326): https://www.antiquity.ac.uk/projgall/kashyap326/

Weber, S. A., Kashyap, A., & Mounce, L. (2006). Archaeobotany at Farmana: new insights into Harappan plant use strategies. Excavations at Farmana, District Rohtak, Haryana,
India, 8, 808-825.

The Ancient Indus Valley Jane R McIntosh http://lukashevichus.info/knigi/

mcintosh_ancient_indus_valley.pdf

Ben-Yehoshua, S., Borowitz, C., & Hanuš, L. O. (2012). Frankincense, myrrh, and balm of Gilead: ancient spices of Southern Arabia and Judea. Horticultural Reviews, Volume 39, 1-76.

Mesopotamian Civilization: The Material Foundations By Daniel T. Potts.

McGovern, P. E., Zhang, J., Tang, J., Zhang, Z., Hall, G. R., Moreau, R. A., ... & Cheng, G. (2004). Fermented beverages of pre-and proto-historic China. Proceedings of the National Academy of Sciences of the United States of America, 101(51), 17593-17598.

David, L. A., Maurice, C. F., Carmody, R. N., Gootenberg, D. B., Button, J. E., Wolfe, B. E., ... & Biddinger, S. B. (2014). Diet rapidly and reproducibly alters the human gut microbiome. Nature, 505(7484), 559.

CHAPTER - GLOBALLY POPULAR AROMATIC PLANTS FROM INDIA

Shinde, V., Deshpande, S., Osada, T., & Uno, T. (2006). Basic issues in Harappan archaeology: Some thoughts. Ancient Asia, 1.

Narayanaswamy, V. (1981). Origin and development of ayurveda:(a brief history). Ancient science of life, 1(1), 1.

Patkar, K. B. (2008). Herbal cosmetics in ancient India. Indian Journal of Plastic Surgery : Official Publication of the Association of Plastic Surgeons of India, 41(Suppl), S134–S137.

SANDALWOOD - incense that helps you relax

Burdock, G. A., & Carabin, I. G. (2008). Safety assessment of sandalwood oil

(Santalum album L.). Food and Chemical Toxicology, 46(2), 421-432.

Bommareddy, A., Rule, B., VanWert, A. L., Santha, S., & Dwivedi, C. (2012). α-Santalol, a derivative of sandalwood oil, induces apoptosis in human prostate cancer cells by causing caspase-3 activation. Phytomedicine, 19(8-9), 804-811.

Santha, S., & Dwivedi, C. (2015). Anticancer effects of sandalwood (Santalum album). Anticancer research, 35(6), 3137-3145.

Ochi, T., Shibata, H., Higuti, T., Kodama, K. H., Kusumi, T., & Takaishi, Y. (2005). Anti-Helicobacter p ylori Compounds from Santalum a lbum. Journal of natural products, 68(6), 819-824.

Schnitzler, P., Koch, C., & Reichling, J. (2007). Susceptibility of drug-resistant clinical herpes simplex virus type 1 strains to essential oils of ginger, thyme, hyssop, and sandalwood. Antimicrobial Agents and Chemotherapy, 51(5), 1859-1862.

Paulpandi, M., Kannan, S., Thangam, R., Kaveri, K., Gunasekaran, P.,

& Rejeeth, C. (2012). In vitro anti-viral effect of β-santalol against influenza viral replication. Phytomedicine, 19(3-4), 231-235.

Heuberger, E., Hongratanaworakit, T., & Buchbauer, G. (2006). East Indian sandalwood and α-santalol odor increase physiological and self-rated arousal in humans. Planta Medica, 72(09), 792-800.

Ahmed, N., Safwan ALI KHAN, M., Manan MAT JAIS, A., Mohtarrudin, N., Ranjbar, M., Shujauddin AMJAD, M., ... & Chincholi, A. (2013). Anti-ulcer activity of sandalwood (Santalum album L.) stem hydro-alcoholic extract in three gastric-ulceration models of wistar rats. Boletín Latinoamericano y del Caribe de Plantas Medicinales y Aromáticas, 12(1).

CAMPHOR - the natural decongestant

Patrick E. McGoverna,1, Armen Mirzoianb, and Gretchen R. Halla aMuseum Applied Science Center for Archaeology, University of Pennsylvania Museum of Archaeology and Anthropology, Philadelphia, PA 19104; and bScientific Services Division, Alcohol and Tobacco Tax and Trade Bureau, U.S. Treasury, Beltsville, MD 20705 Edited by Ofer Bar-Yosef, Harvard University, Cambridge, MA, and approved February 23, 2009

I, H., Huang, L., Zhou, A., Li, X., & Sun, J. (2009). Study on antiinflammatory effect of different chemotype of Cinnamomum camphora on rat arthritis model induced by Freund's

adjuvant. Zhongguo Zhong yao za zhi= Zhongguo zhongyao zazhi= China journal of Chinese materia medica, 34(24), 3251-3254.

Liu, L., Wei, F. X., Qu, Z. Y., Wang, S. Q., Chen, G., Gao, H., & Wang, Y. C. (2009). The antiadenovirus activities of cinnamaldehyde in vitro. Laboratory Medicine, 40(11), 669-674.

Pragadheesh, V. S., Saroj, A., Yadav, A., Chanotiya, C. S., Alam, M., & Samad, A. (2013). Chemical characterization and antifungal activity of Cinnamomum camphora essential oil. Industrial crops and products, 49, 628-633.

Frizzo, C. D., Santos, A. C., Paroul, N., Serafini, L. A., Dellacassa, E.,

Lorenzo, D., & Moyna, P. (2000). Essential oils of camphor tree (cinnamomum camphora nees & eberm) cultivated in Southern Brazil. Brazilian Archives of Biology and Technology, 43(3), 313-316.

Rabadia, J., Satish, S., Ramanjaneyulu, J., & Narayanaswamy, V. B. (2013). An Investigation of Anti-Depressant Activity of Cinnamomum Camphora Oil in Experimental Mice. Asian Journal of Biomedical and Pharmaceutical Sciences, 3(20), 44.

Jadhav, M. V., Sharma, R. C., & Rathore Mansee, G. A. (2010). Effect

of Cinnamomum camphora on human sperm motility and sperm viability. J Clin Res Lett, 1(1), 01-10.

Chen, W., Vermaak, I., & Viljoen, A. (2013). Camphor—a fumigant

during the black death and a coveted fragrant wood in ancient Egypt and Babylon—a review. Molecules, 18(5), 5434-5454.

HOLY BASIL- the miracle medicinal plant

Gupta, P., Yadav, D. K., Siripurapu, K. B., Palit, G., & Maurya, R. (2007). Constituents of Ocimum sanctum with antistress activity. Journal of natural products, 70(9), 1410-1416.

Hakkim, F. L., Shankar, C. G., & Girija, S. (2007). Chemical composition and antioxidant property of holy basil (Ocimum sanctum L.) leaves, stems, and inflorescence and their in vitro callus cultures. Journal of agricultural and food chemistry, 55(22), 9109-9117.

Geetha, R. K., & Vasudevan, D. M. (2004). Inhibition of lipid peroxidation by botanical extracts of Ocimum sanctum: in vivo and in vitro studies. Life sciences, 76(1), 21-28.
Manikandan, P., Murugan, R. S., Abbas, H., Abraham, S. K.,

&   Nagini, S. (2007). Ocimum sanctum Linn.(holy basil) ethanolic leaf extract protects against 7, 12-dimethylbenz [a] anthracene-induced genotoxicity, oxidative stress, and imbalance in xenobiotic-metabolizing enzymes. Journal of medicinal food, 10(3), 495-502.

Subramanian, M., Chintalwar, G. J., & Chattopadhyay, S. (2005). Antioxidant and radioprotective properties of an Ocimum sanctum polysaccharide. Redox

Report, 10(5), 257-264.

Samson, J., Sheeladevi, R., & Ravindran, R. (2007). Oxidative stress in brain and antioxidant activity of Ocimum sanctum in noise exposure. Neurotoxicology, 28(3), 679-685.

Muthuraman, A., Diwan, V., Jaggi, A. S., Singh, N., & Singh, D. (2008). Ameliorative effects of Ocimum sanctum in sciatic nerve transection-induced neuropathy in rats. Journal of ethnopharmacology, 120(1), 56-62.

Archana, R., & Namasivayam, A. (2002). A comparative study of different crude extracts of Ocimum sanctum on noise stress. Phytotherapy Research, 16(6), 579-580.

Samson, J., Devi, R. S., Ravindran, R., & Senthilvelan, M. (2006). Biogenic amine changes in brain regions and attenuating action of Ocimum sanctumin noise exposure. Pharmacology Biochemistry and Behavior, 83(1), 67-75.

Ravindran, R., Devi, R. S., Samson, J., & Senthilvelan, M. (2005). Noise-stress-induced brain neurotransmitter changes and the effect of Ocimum sanctum (Linn) treatment in albino rats. Journal of pharmacological sciences, 98(4), 354-360.

Khanna, N., & Bhatia, J. (2003). Antinociceptive action of Ocimum sanctum (Tulsi) in mice: possible mechanisms involved. Journal of ethnopharmacology, 88(2-3), 293-296.

Yanpallewar, S. U., Rai, S., Kumar, M., & Acharya, S. B. (2004). Evaluation of antioxidant and neuroprotective effect of Ocimum sanctum on transient cerebral ischemia and long-term cerebral hypoperfusion. Pharmacology Biochemistry and Behavior, 79(1), 155-164.

Kapoor, S. (2008). Ocimum sanctum: A therapeutic role in diabetes and the metabolic syndrome. Hormone and metabolic research, 40(04), 296-296.

Reddy, S. S., Karuna, R., Baskar, R., & Saralakumari, D. (2008). Prevention of insulin resistance by ingesting aqueous extract of Ocimum sanctum to fructose-fed rats. Hormone and Metabolic Research, 40(01), 44-49.

Vats, V., Yadav, S. P., & Grover, J. K. (2004). Ethanolic extract of Ocimum sanctum leaves partially attenuates streptozotocin-induced alterations in glycogen content and carbohydrate metabolism in rats. Journal of ethnopharmacology, 90(1), 155-160.

Hannan, J. M. A., Marenah, L., Ali, L., Rokeya, B., Flatt, P. R., & Abdel-Wahab, Y. H. A. (2006). Ocimum sanctum leaf extracts stimulate insulin secretion from perfused pancreas, isolated islets and clonal pancreatic β-cells. Journal of Endocrinology, 189(1), 127-136.

Shokeen, P., Bala, M., Singh, M., & Tandon, V. (2008). In vitro activity of eugenol, an active component from Ocimum sanctum, against multiresistant and susceptible strains of Neisseria gonorrhoeae. International journal of antimicrobial agents, 32(2), 174-179.

Shokeen, P., Ray, K., Bala, M., & Tandon, V. (2005). Preliminary studies on activity of Ocimum sanctum, Drynaria quercifolia, and Annona squamosa against Neisseria gonorrhoeae. Sexually transmitted diseases, 32(2), 106-111.

Nayak, V., & Devi, P. U. (2005). Protection of mouse bone marrow

against radiation-induced chromosome damage and stem cell death by the ocimum flavonoids orientin and vicenin. Radiation research, 163(2), 165-171.

Siddique, Y., Ara, G., Beg, T., & Afzal, M. (2007). Anti-genotoxic effect of Ocimum sanctum L. extract against cyproterone acetate induced genotoxic damage in cultured mammalian cells. Acta Biologica Hungarica, 58(4), 397-409.

Dutta, D. I. P. A. N. W. I. T. A., Devi, S. S., Krishnamuthi, K., Kumar, K., Vyas, P., Muthal, P. L., … & Chakrabarti, T. (2007). Modulatory effect of distillate of Ocimum sanctum leaf extract (Tulsi) on human lymphocytes against genotoxicants. Biomedical and Environmental Sciences, 20(3), 226.

Manikandan, P., Prathiba, D., & Nagini, S. (2007). Proliferation, angiogenesis and apoptosis-associated proteins are molecular targets for chemoprevention of MNNG-induced gastric carcinogenesis by ethanolic Ocimum sanctum leaf extract. Singapore medical journal, 48(7), 645-651.

Rastogi, S., Shukla, Y., Paul, B. N., Chowdhuri, D. K., Khanna, S. K., & Das, M. (2007). Protective effect of Ocimum sanctum on 3-methylcholanthrene, 7, 12-dimethylbenz (a) anthracene and aflatoxin B1 induced skin tumorigenesis in mice. Toxicology and applied pharmacology, 224(3), 228-240.

Dharmani, P., Kuchibhotla, V. K., Maurya, R., Srivastava, S., Sharma, S., & Palit, G. (2004). Evaluation of anti-ulcerogenic and ulcer-healing properties of Ocimum sanctum Linn. Journal of ethnopharmacology, 93(2-3), 197-206.

Goel, R. K., Sairam, K., Dorababu, M., Prabha, T., & Rao, C. V. (2005). Effect of standardized extract of Ocimum sanctum Linn. on gastric mucosal offensive and defensive factors.

Kath, R. K., & Gupta, R. K. (2006). Antioxidant activity of hydroalcoholic leaf extract of Ocimum sanctum in animal models of peptic ulcer. Indian journal of physiology and pharmacology, 50(4), 391.

Singh, S., & Majumdar, D. K. (1999). Evaluation of the gastric antiulcer activity of fixed oil of Ocimum sanctum (Holy Basil). Journal of ethnopharmacology, 65(1), 13-19.

Sood, S., Narang, D., Thomas, M. K., Gupta, Y. K., & Maulik, S. K. (2006). Effect of Ocimum sanctum Linn. on cardiac changes in rats subjected to chronic restraint stress. Journal of ethnopharmacology, 108(3), 423-427.

Mohanty, I., Arya, D. S., & Gupta, S. K. (2006). Effect of Curcuma longa and Ocimum sanctum on myocardial apoptosis in experimentally induced myocardial ischemic-reperfusion injury. BMC complementary and alternative medicine, 6(1), 3.

Ahmed, M., Ahamed, R. N., Aladakatti, R. H., & Ghosesawar, M. G. (2002). Reversible anti-fertility effect of benzene extract of Ocimum sanctum leaves on sperm parameters and fructose content in rats. Journal of basic and clinical physiology and pharmacology, 13(1), 51-60.

Gupta, S. K., Prakash, J., & Srivastava, S. (2002). Validation of traditional claim of Tulsi, Ocimum sanctum Linn. as a medicinal plant.

Devi, P. U. (2001). Radioprotective, anticarcinogenic and antioxidant properties of the Indian holy basil, Ocimum sanctum (Tulasi).

Ballal, M. (2001). Activity of Ocimum sanctum (the traditional Indian medicinal plant) against the enteric pathogens. Indian Journal of Medical Sciences, 55(8), 434-438.

Prakash, J., & Gupta, S. K. (2000). Chemopreventive activity of Ocimum sanctum seed oil. Journal of ethnopharmacology, 72(1-2), 29-34.

Agrawal, P., Rai, V., & Singh, R. B. (1996). Randomized placebo-controlled, single blind trial of holy basil leaves in patients with noninsulin-dependent diabetes mellitus. International journal of clinical pharmacology and therapeutics, 34(9), 406-409.

Sembulingam, K., Sembulingam, P., & Namasivayam, A. (2005). Effect of Ocimum sanctum Linn on the changes in central cholinergic system induced by acute noise stress. Journal of ethnopharmacology, 96(3), 477-482.

Sembulingam, K., Sembulingam, P., & Namasivayam, A. (1997). Effect of Ocimum sanctum Linn on noise induced changes in plasma corticosterone level. Indian journal of physiology and pharmacology, 41, 139-143.

Archana, R., & Namasivayam, A. (2000). Effect of Ocimum sanctum on noise induced changes in neutrophil functions. Journal of ethnopharmacology, 73(1-2), 81-85.

Sen, P., Maiti, P. C., Puri, S., Ray, A., Audulov, N. A., & Valdman, A. V. (1992). Mechanism of anti-stress activity of Ocimum sanctum Linn, eugenol and Tinospora malabarica in experimental animals. Indian journal of experimental biology, 30(7), 592-596.

CHAPTER - INDIAN SACRED TREES

Khan, M. L., Khumbongmayum, A. D., & Tripathi, R. S. (2008). The sacred groves and their significance in conserving biodiversity: an overview. International Journal of Ecology and Environmental Sciences, 34(3), 277-291.

Ray, R., Chandran, M. D. S., & Ramachandra, T. V. (2014). Biodiversity and ecological assessments of Indian sacred groves. Journal of forestry research, 25(1), 21-28.

Ficus religiosa - the tree that Hindus workship

Makhija, I. K., Sharma, I. P., & Khamar, D. (2010). Phytochemistry and Pharmacological properties of Ficus religiosa: an overview. Ann Biol Res, 1(4), 171-180.

Gulecha, V., Sivakumar, T., Upaganlawar, A., Mahajan, M., & Upasani, C. (2011). Screening of Ficus religiosa leaves fractions for analgesic and anti-inflammatory activities. Indian journal of pharmacology, 43(6), 662.

Ahuja, D., Bijjem, K. R. V., & Kalia, A. N. (2011). Bronchospasm potentiating effect of methanolic extract of Ficus religiosa fruits in guinea pigs. Journal of ethnopharmacology, 133(2), 324-328.

Devi, W. B., Sengottuvela, S., Haja, S. S., Lalitha, V., & Sivakumar, T. (2011). Memory enhancing activities of Ficus religiosa leaves in rodents. International Journal of Research in Ayurveda and Pharmacy, 2(3), 834-838.

Hamed, M. A. (2011). Beneficial effect of Ficus religiosa Linn. on high-fat-diet-induced hypercholesterolemia in rats. Food chemistry, 129(1), 162-170.

Kaur, H., Singh, D., Singh, B., & Goel, R. K. (2010). Anti-amnesic effect of Ficus religiosa in scopolamine-induced anterograde and retrograde amnesia. Pharmaceutical biology, 48(2), 234-240.

Khan, M. S. A., Hussain, S. A., Jais, A. M. M., Zakaria, Z. A., & Khan, M. (2011). Anti-ulcer activity of Ficus religiosa stem bark ethanolic extract in rats. Journal of Medicinal Plants Research, 5(3), 354-359.

Pandit, R., Phadke, A., & Jagtap, A. (2010). Antidiabetic effect of Ficus religiosa extract in streptozotocin-induced diabetic rats. Journal of ethnopharmacology, 128(2), 462-466.

Patil M. S., Patil, M. S., Patil, C. R., Patil, S. W., & Jadhav, R. B. (2011). Anticonvulsant activity of aqueous root extract of Ficus religiosa. Journal of ethnopharmacology, 133(1), 92-96.

Prasad, P. V., Subhaktha, P. K., Narayana, A., & Rao, M. M. (2006). Medico-historical study of "aśvattha" (sacred fig tree). Bulletin of the Indian Institute of History of Medicine (Hyderabad), 36(1), 1-20.

Roy, K., Shivakumar, H., & Sarkar, S. (2009). Wound healing potential of leaf extracts of Ficus religiosa on Wistar albino strain rats. Int J Pharm Tech Res, 1, 506-8.

Saha, S., & Goswami, G. (2010). Study of anti ulcer activity of Ficus religiosa

L. on experimentally induced gastric ulcers in rats. Asian Pacific Journal of Tropical Medicine, 3(10), 791-793.

Singh, D., & Goel, R. K. (2009). Anticonvulsant effect of Ficus religiosa: role of serotonergic pathways. Journal of ethnopharmacology, 123(2), 330-334.

Sreelekshmi, R., Latha, P. G., Arafat, M. M., Arafat, M. M., Shyamal, S., Shine, V. J., ... & Rajasekharan, S. (2007). Anti-inflammatory, analgesic and anti-lipid peroxidation studies on stem bark of Ficus religiosa Linn.

Viswanathan, S., Thirugnanasambantham, P., Reddy, M. K., Narasimhan, S., & Subramaniam, G. A. (1990). Anti-inflammatory and mast cell protective effect of Ficus religiosa. Ancient science of life, 10(2), 122.

Verma, N., Chaudhary, S., Garg, V. K., & Tyagi, S. (2010). Antiinflammatory and analgesic activity of methanolic extract of stem bark of Ficus religiosa. International Journal of Pharma Professional's Research, 1(2), 145.

Yadav, Y. C., Srivastava, D. N., Saini, V., Sighal, S., Kumar, S., Seth, K. A., & Ghelani, K. T. (2011). Experimental Studies of Ficus religiosa (L) latex for preventive and curative effect against cisplatin induced nephrotoxicity in wistar rats. J Chem Pharm Res, 3(1), 621-7.

Ficus benghalensis - tree with a thousand trunks

Garg, V. K., & Paliwal, S. K. (2011). Wound-healing activity of ethanolic and aqueous extracts of Ficus benghalensis. Journal of advanced pharmaceutical technology & research, 2(2), 110.

Patel, M. A., Patel, P. K., & Patel, M. B. (2010). Effects of ethanol extract of Ficus bengalensis (bark) on inflammatory bowel disease. Indian journal of pharmacology, 42(4), 214.

Gabhe, S. Y., Tatke, P. A., & Khan, T. A. (2006). Evaluation of the immunomodulatory activity of the methanol extract of Ficus benghalensis roots in rats. Indian journal of pharmacology, 38(4), 271.

Deshmukh, V. K., Shrotri, D. S., & Aiman, R. (1960). Isolation of a hypoglycemic principle from the bark of Ficus bengalensis Linn. A preliminary note. Indian journal of physiology and pharmacology, 4, 182-185.

Shukla, R., Gupta, S., Gambhir, J. K., Prabhu, K. M., & Murthy, P. S. (2004). Antioxidant effect of aqueous extract of the bark of Ficus bengalensis in hypercholesterolaemic rabbits. Journal of ethnopharmacology, 92(1), 47-51.

Taur, D. J., Nirmal, S. A., Patil, R. Y., & Kharya, M. D. (2007). Antistress and antiallergic effects of Ficus bengalensis bark in asthma. Natural product research, 21(14), 1266-1270.

Aswar, M., Aswar, U., Watkar, B., Vyas, M., Wagh, A., & Gujar, K. N. (2008). Anthelmintic activity of Ficus benghalensis. International Journal of Green Pharmacy (IJGP), 2(3).

Augusti, K. T. (1975). Hypoglycaemic action of bengalenoside, a glucoside isolated from Ficus bengalensis Linn, in normal and alloxan diabetic rabbits. Indian journal of physiology and pharmacology, 19(4), 218-220.

Murti, K., & Kumar, U. (2011). Antimicrobial activity of Ficus benghalensis and Ficus racemosa roots L. Am. J. Microbiol, 2(1), 21-24.

Satish, A., Kumar, R. P., Rakshith, D., Satish, S., & Ahmed, F. (2013). Antimutagenic and antioxidant activity of Ficus benghalensis stem bark and Moringa oleifera root extract. International Journal of Chemical and Analytical Science, 4(2), 45-48.

Gaherwal, S. (2013). Anti-bacterial activity of ficus benghalensis (Banyan) fruit extract against difffrent bacteria. International Journal of Microbiological Research, 4(2), 177-179.

Deore, A. B., Mule, S. N., & Sapakal, V. D. (2012). Evaluation of Anti-inflammatory Activity of Ficus benghalensis in Rats. Journal of Biologically Active Products from Nature, 2(2), 85-89.

AEGLE MARMELOS fruits that tone the digestinve system

Nigam, V., & Nambiar, V. International Journal of Ayurvedic and Herbal Medicine 4: 6 (2014) 1634-1648.

Ariharan, V. N., & Nagendra Prasad, P. (2013). Mahavilva-a sacred tree with immense medicinal secrets: a mini review. Rasayan J Chemistry, 6(4), 342-352.

Baliga, M. S., Bhat, H. P., Joseph, N., & Fazal, F. (2011). Phytochemistry and medicinal uses of the bael fruit (Aegle marmelos Correa): A concise review. Food Research International, 44(7), 1768-1775.

Sekar, D. K., Kumar, G., Karthik, L., & Rao, K. B. (2011). A review on pharmacological and phytochemical properties of Aegle marmelos (L.) Corr. Serr.(Rutaceae). Asian Journal of Plant Science and Research, 1(2), 8-17.

Sharma, G. N., Dubey, S. K., Sati, N., & Sanadya, J. (2011). Anti-inflammatory activity and total flavonoid content of Aegle marmelos seeds. Int J Pharm Sci Drug Res, 3(3), 214-8.

Rajan, S., Gokila, M., Jency, P., Brindha, P., & Sujatha, R. K. (2011). Antioxidant and phytochemical properties of Aegle marmelos fruit pulp. International journal of current pharmaceutical research, 3(2), 65-70.

Sharma, G. N., Dubey, S. K., Sati, N., & Sanadya, J. (2011). Ulcer healing potential of Aegle marmelos fruit seed. Asian J Pharm Life Sci, 1(2), 172-178.

Pandey, A., & Mishra, R. (2011). Antibacterial properties of Aegle marmelos leaves, fruits and peels against various pathogens. Journal of

Pharmaceutical and Biomedical Sciences, 13(13).

Kaur, P., Walia, A., Kumar, S., & Kaur, S. (2009). Antigenotoxic activity of polyphenolic rich extracts from Aegle marmelos (L.) Correa in human blood lymphocytes and E. coli PQ 37. Records of Natural Products, 3(1), 68.

Upadhya, S., Shanbhag, K. K., Suneetha, G., Balachandra Naidu, M.,

& Upadhya, S. (2004). A study of hypoglycemic and antioxidant activity of Aegle marmelos in alloxan induced diabetic rats. Indian J Physiol Pharmacol, 48(4), 476-480.

Jayachandra, K., & Sivaraman, T. (2011). Hepatoprotective Effect of Aegle Marmelos (L.) Corr. Leaf Powder (Crude) Against Carbon Tetrachloride-Induced Hepatic Damage in Albino Rats. Journal of Pharmaceutical Sciences and Research, 3(7), 1360-1363.

Singh, K., Agrawal, K. K., & Gupta, J. K. (2012). Comparative anthelmintic activity of Aegle marmelos Linn leaves and pulp. IOSR/Journal of Pharmacy, 2(3), 395-397.

Das, S. W. A. R. N. A. M. O. N. I., Hakim, A. B. D. U. L., & Mittal, A. J. A. Y. (2012). Study of the antihyperlipidemic, antioxidative and antiatherogenic activity of Aegle marmelos linn. in rabbit receiving high fat diet. Asian j pharm clin res, 5(4), 69-72.

Anthocephalus kadamba with flowers for lovers

Mishra, R. P. (2011). Antibacterial Properties of Anthocephalus Cadamba Fruits.

Acharyya, S., Dash, G. K., Mondal, S., & Dash, S. K. (2010). Studies on glucose lowering efficacy of the Anthocephalus cadamba (Roxb.) Miq. roots. International Journal of Pharma and Bio Sciences, 1(2).

DUBEY, A., Nayak, S., & Goupale, D. C. (2011). DEVELOPMENT AND EVALUATION OF ANTIMICROBIAL FORMULATION CONTAINING EXTRACT OF ANTHOCEPHALUS CADAMBA (ROXB.) MIQ. LEAVES. Int. J. Pharm. Res. Dev., 3, 8-12.

Alam, M. A., Subhan, N., Chowdhury, S. A., Awal, M. A., Mostofa, M., Rashid, M. A., ... & Sarker, S. D. (2011). Anthocephalus cadamba (Roxb.) Miq., Rubiaceae, extract shows hypoglycemic effect and eases oxidative stress in alloxan-induced diabetic rats. Revista Brasileira de Farmacognosia, 21(1), 0-0.

Usman, M. R. M., Somani, R. P., Mohammed, A., & Mohammed, U. (2012). Evaluation of antipyretic activity of Anthocephalus cadamba roxb. leaves extracts. Res J Pharm Biol Chem Sci, 3(1), 825-34.

Chandrashekar, K. S., Abinash, B., & Prasanna, K. S. (2010). Anti-inflammatory effect of the methanol extract from Anthocephalus cadamba stem bark in animal modelsa. International Journal of Plant Biology, 1(1).

Singh, S., Ishar, M. P. S., Saxena, A. K., & Kaur, A. (2013). Cytotoxic effect of Anthocephalus cadamba Miq. leaves on human cancer cell lines. Pharmacognosy Journal, 5(3), 127-129.

Nagakannan, P., Shivasharan, B. D., Veerapur, V. P., & Thippeswamy, B. S. (2011). Sedative and antiepileptic effects of Anthocephalus cadamba Roxb. in mice and rats. Indian journal of pharmacology, 43(6), 699.

ASOKA- Saraca asoca

Verma, A., Jana, G. K., Sen, S., Chakraborty, R., Sachan, S., & Mishra, A. (2010). Pharmacological evaluation of Saraca indica leaves for central nervous system depressant activity in mice. J Pharm Sci Res, 2(6), 338-343.

Sharma, A., Gupta, S., Sachan, S., Mishra, A., & Banarji, A. (2011).

Anthelmintic activity of the leaf of Saraca indica Linn. Asian Journal of Pharmacy and Life Science ISSN, 2231, 4423.

Swamy, A. V., Patel, U. M., Koti, B. C., Gadad, P. C., Patel, N. L., & Thippeswamy, A. H. M. (2013). Cardioprotective effect of Saraca indica against cyclophosphamide induced cardiotoxicity in rats: A biochemical, electrocardiographic and histopathological study. Indian journal of pharmacology, 45(1), 44.

Asokan, A., & Thangavel, M. (2014). In vitro cytotoxic studies of crude methanolic extract of Saracaindica bark extract, IOSR J. Pharm. Biol. Sci, 9, 26-30.

Sarojini, N., Manjari, S. A., & Kanti, C. C. (2011). Phytochemical screening and antibacterial activity study of Saraca indica leaves extract. Int. Res. J. Pharm, 2, 176-179.

Verma, A., Jana, G. K., Chakraborty, R., Sen, S., Sachan, S., & Mishra, A. (2010). Analgesic activity of various leaf extracts of Saraca indica Linn. Der Pharmacia Lettre, 2(3), 35.

Panchawat, S., & Sisodia, S. S. (2010). In vitro antioxidant activity of Saraca asoca Roxb. De Wilde stem bark extracts from various extraction processes. Asian J. Pharm. Clin. Res, 3(3).

Panchawat, S., & Sisodia, S. S. (2011). In-vivo antidiarrhoeal activity of extracts from stem bark of Saraca asoca Roxb. prepared by different extraction methods. Indent, 166(113548).

Elaeocarpus ganitrus with psychotherapeutic fruits

Garg, K. A. L. P. A. N. A., Goswami, K. O. M. A. L., & Khurana, G. A. U. R. A. V. (2013). A pharmacognostical review on Elaeocarpus sphaericus. Int J Pharm Pharm Sci, 5(1), 3-8.

Sarma, J. K., & Bhuyan, G. C. (2004). An experimental evaluation of the effect of rudraksha (Elaeocarpus ganitrus roxb) in adrenaline and nicotine induced hypertension. Ancient science of life, 23(4), 1.

Sakat, S. S., Wankhede, S. S., Juvekar, A. R., Mali, V. R., & Bodhankar, S. L. (2009). Antihypertensive effect of aqueous extract of Elaeocarpus ganitrus Roxb. seeds in renal artery occluded hypertensive rats. International Journal of PharmTech Research, 1(3), 779-782.

Rao, K. S., Rao, O. U., Aminabee, S. K., Rao, C. R. M., & Rao, A. L. (2012). Hypoglycemic and antidiabetic potential of chitosan aqueous extract of Elaeocarpus ganitrus. International journal of research in pharmacy and chemistry, 2(2), 428-441.

Hule, A. K., Shah, A. S., Gambhire, M. N., & Juvekar, A. R. (2011). An evaluation of the antidiabetic effects of Elaeocarpus ganitrus in experimental animals. Indian journal of pharmacology, 43(1), 56.

Rashmi, P., & Amrinder, K. (2014). Mythological and Spiritual Review on Eloeocarpus Ganitrus and Assessment of Scientific Facts for its Medicinal Uses. International Journal of Research, 1(5), 334-353.

Rauniar, G. P., & Sharma, M. (2012). Evaluation of anxiolytic effect of elaeocarpus ganitrus in mice. Health Renaissance, 10(2), 108-112.

Singh, B., Chopra, A., Ishar, M. P. S., Sharma, A., & Raj, T. (2010). Pharmacognostic and antifungal investigations of Elaeocarpus ganitrus (Rudrakasha). Indian journal of pharmaceutical sciences, 72(2), 261.

Sathish Kumar, T., Shanmugam, S., Palvannan, T., & Bharathi Kumar, V. M. (2010). Evaluation of antioxidant properties of Elaeocarpus ganitrus Roxb. leaves. Iranian Journal of Pharmaceutical Research, 211-215.

Kumar, G., Karthik, L., & Rao, K. V. B. (2011). Antimicrobial activity of Elaeocarpus ganitrus Roxb (Elaeocarpaceae): An in vitro study.

MANGO, the King of Indian fruits

Shah, K. A., Patel, M. B., Patel, R. J., & Parmar, P. K. (2010). Mangifera indica (mango). Pharmacognosy reviews, 4(7), 42.

Chaisawadi, S., Suwanyeun, S., & Boonnumma, S. (2011, December).

Freeze-dried mango powder processing for nutraceutical use. In International Symposium on Medicinal and Aromatic Plants 1023 (pp. 95-100).

Wauthoz, N., Balde, A., Balde, E. S., Van Damme, M., & Duez, P. (2007). Ethnopharmacology of Mangifera indica L. bark and pharmacological studies of its main C-glucosylxanthone, mangiferin. International Journal of Biomedical and Pharmaceutical Sciences, 1(2), 112-119.

Kemasari, P., Sangeetha, S., & Venkatalakshmi, P. (2011). Antihyperglycemic activity of Mangifera indica Linn. in alloxan induced diabetic rats. J Chem Pharm Res, 3(5), 653-9.

Joona, K., Sowmia, C., Dhanya, K. P., & Divya, M. J. (2013). Preliminary Phytochemical Investigation of Mangifera indica leaves and screening of Antioxidant and Anticancer activity. Research journal of pharmaceutical, biological and chemical sciences, 4(1), 1112-1118.

El-Gied, A. A. A., Joseph, M. R., Mahmoud, I. M., Abdelkareem, A. M., Al Hakami, A. M., & Hamid, M. E. (2012). Antimicrobial activities of seed extracts of mango (Mangifera indica L.). Advances in Microbiology, 2(1), 571-576.

Doughari, J. H., & Manzara, S. (2008). In vitro antibacterial activity of crude leaf extracts of Mangifera indica Linn. African journal of Microbiology research, 2(1), 67-72.

Olorunfemi, O. J., Nworah, D. C., Egwurugwu, J. N., & Hart, V. O. (2012). Evaluation of anti-inflammatory, analgesic and antipyretic effect of Mangifera indica leaf extract on fever-induced albino rats (Wistar). British Journal of Pharmacology and Toxicology, 3(2), 54-57.

Jiang, Y., You, X. Y., Fu, K. L., & Yin, W. L. (2012). Effects of extract from Mangifera indica leaf on monosodium urate crystal-induced gouty arthritis in rats. Evidence-Based Complementary and Alternative Medicine, 2012.

Naved, T., Siddiqui, J. I., Ansari, S. H., Ansari, A. A., & Mukhtar, H.

M. (2005). Immunomodulatory activity of Mangifera indica L.
fruits (cv Neelam). Journal of Natural Remedies, 5(2), 137-140.

Neelima, N., Sudhakar, M., Patil, M. B., & Lakshmi, B. V. S. (2017). Anti-ulcer activity and HPTLC analysis of Mangifera indica L. leaves. International Journal of Pharmaceutical and Phytopharmacological Research, 1(4), 146-155.

Kittiphoom, S., & Sutasinee, S. (2013). Mango seed kernel oil and its physicochemical properties. Int Food Res J, 20(3), 1145-1149.

Dhananjaya, B. L., Zameer, F., Girish, K. S., & DSouza, C. J. (2011). Anti-venom potential of aqueous extract of stem bark of Mangifera indica L. against Daboia russellii (Russell's viper) venom.

García-Rivera, D., Delgado, R., Bougarne, N., Haegeman, G.,

& Berghe, W. V. (2011). Gallic acid indanone and mangiferin xanthone are strong determinants of immunosuppressive anti-tumour effects of Mangifera indica L. bark in MDA-MB231 breast cancer cells. Cancer letters, 305(1), 21-31.

AZADIRACHTA INDICA- the natural antibiotic

Hashmat, I., Azad, H., & Ahmed, A. (2012). Neem (Azadirachta indica A. Juss)-A nature's drugstore: an overview. Int Res J Biol Sci, 1(6), 76-79.

Awofeso, N. (2011). Neem tree extract Azadirachta indica and malaria control in Africa and Asia: prospects and challenges. Spatula DD-Tamamlayıcı Tıp ve İlaç Geliştirme Alanında Hakemli Dergi, 1(3), 167-174.

Bedri, S., Khalil, E. A., Khalid, S. A., Alzohairy, M. A., Mohieldein, A., Aldebasi, Y. H., ... & Farahna, M. (2013). Azadirachta indica ethanolic extract protects neurons from apoptosis and mitigates brain swelling in experimental cerebral malaria. Malaria journal, 12(1), 298.

Habluetzel, A., Lucantoni, L., & Esposito, F. (2009). Azadirachta indica as a public health tool for the control of malaria & other vector-borne diseases.

Nayak, B. R., Rao, N. M., & Pattabiraman, T. N. (1979). Studies on plant gums. Proteases in neem (Azadirachta indica) gum. Journal of Biosciences, 1(4), 393-400.

Chatterjee, A., Saluja, M., Singh, N., & Kandwal, A. (2011). To evaluate the antigingivitis and antipalque effect of an Azadirachta indica (neem) mouthrinse on plaque induced gingivitis: A double-blind, randomized, controlled trial. Journal of Indian Society of Periodontology, 15(4), 398.

Boadu, K. O., Tulashie, S. K., Anang, M. A., & Kpan, J. D. (2011). Production of natural insecticide from Neem leaves (Azadirachta indica). Asian J. Plant. Sci. Res, 1(4), 33-38.

Kato-Noguchi, H., Salam, M. A., Ohno, O., & Suenaga, K. (2014). Nimbolide B and Nimbic Acid B, phytotoxic substances in neem leaves with allelopathic activity. Molecules, 19(6), 6929-6940.

Imran, K., Srikakolupu, S. R., Surekha, D., Gotteti, S. D., & Hemasundara, A. (2010). Phytochemical studies and screening of leaf extracts of Azadirachta indica for its anti-microbial activity against dental pathogens. Archives of Applied Science Research, 2(2), 246-250.

Khosla, P., Bhanwra, S. A. N. G. E. E. T. A., Singh, J., Seth, S.,

& Srivastava, R. K. (2000). A study of hypoglycaemic effects of Azadirachta indica (Neem) in normal and alloxan diabetic rabbits. Indian Journal of Physiology and Pharmacology, 44(1), 69-74.

Schmutterer, H. (1990). Properties and potential of natural pesticides from the neem tree, Azadirachta indica. Annual review of entomology, 35(1), 271-297.

Sharma, T., & Khan, A. M. (2008). Toxic effect of neem (Azadirachta indica) extracts against Schistocerca gregaria F. adults under laboratory conditions. J. Environ. Res. Develop, 2(4).

Grover, A., Bhandari, B. S., & Rai, N. (2011). Antimicrobial activity of medicinal plants-Azadirachta indica A. Juss, Allium cepa L. and Aloe vera L. Int J Pharm Tech Res, 3, 1059-1065.

Raghavendra, M., Maiti, R., Kumar, S., & Acharya, S. B. (2013). Role of aqueous extract of Azadirachta indica leaves in an experimental model of Alzheimer's disease in rats. International Journal of Applied and Basic Medical Research, 3(1), 37.

Khan, S., Halim, S. A., Kashif, M., Jabeen, A., Asif, M., Mesaik, M. A., ... & Choudhary, M. I. (2013). In-vitro immunomodulatory and anti-cancerous activities of biotransformed products of Dianabol through Azadirachta indica and its molecular docking studies. Chemistry Central Journal, 7(1), 163.

Al-Hazmi, R. H. M. (2013). Effect of Neem (Azadirachta indica) leaves and seeds extract on the growth of six of the plant disease causing fungi. Global

Advanced Research Journal of Microbiology, 2(5), 089-098.

Nand, P., Drabu, S., & Gupta, R. K. (2012). Insignificant anti-acne activity of Azadirachta indica leaves and bark. Journal of Pharmaceutical Negative Results, 3(1), 29.

Bharitkar, Y. P., Bathini, S., Ojha, D., Ghosh, S., Mukherjee, H., Kuotsu, K., … & Mondal, N. B. (2014). Antibacterial and antiviral evaluation of sulfonoquinovosyldiacylglyceride: a glycolipid isolated from Azadirachta indica leaves. Letters in applied microbiology, 58(2), 184-189.

Aladakatti, R. H., & Ahamed, R. N. (2006). Azadirachta indica A. Juss induced changes in spermatogenic pattern in albino rats. Journal of Natural Remedies, 6(1), 62-72.

Akhtar, M. (2000). Nematicidal potential of the neem tree Azadirachta indica (A. Juss). Integrated Pest Management Reviews, 5(1), 57-66.

Nicoletti, M., Maccioni, O., Coccioletti, T., Mariani, S., & Vitali, F. (2012). Neem tree (Azadirachta indica A. Juss) as source of bioinsectides. In Insecticides-Advances in Integrated Pest Management. InTech.

Shailey, S., & Basir, S. F. (2012). Strengthening of antioxidant defense by Azadirachta indica in alloxan-diabetic rat tissues. Journal of Ayurveda and integrative medicine, 3(3), 130.

Lloyd, A. C., Menon, T., & Umamaheshwari, K. (2005). Anticandidal activity of Azadirachta indica. Indian journal of Pharmacology, 37(6), 386.

Geraldo, M. R. F., Arroteia, C. C., & Kemmelmeier, C. (2010). The effects of neem [Azadirachta indica A. Juss (meliaceae)] oil on Fusarium oxysporum f. sp. medicagenis and Fusarium subglutinans and the production of fusaric acid toxin. Advances in Bioscience and Biotechnology, 1(01), 1.

Satti, A. A., Elamin, M. M., & Futuwi, A. I. (2013). Insecticidal effects of neem (Azadirachta indica A. Juss) oils obtained from neem berries stored at different periods. The Experiment, 6(2), 330-337.

Chourasiya, A., Upadhaya, A., & Shukla, R. N. (2012). Isolation of quercetin-from leaves of Azadirachta Indica and anti-diabetic study of the crude extracts. Journal of pharmaceutical and biomedical science, 25, 179-181.

Siddiqui, B. S., Rasheed, M., Ilyas, F., Gulzar, T., Tariq, R. M., & Naqvi, S. N. U. H. (2004). Analysis of insecticidal Azadirachta indica A. Juss. fractions. Zeitschrift für Naturforschung C, 59(1-2), 104-112.

Boadu, K. O., Tulashie, S. K., Anang, M. A., & Kpan, J. D. (2011). Production of natural insecticide from Neem leaves (Azadirachta indica). Asian J. Plant. Sci. Res, 1(4), 33-38.

Kaushik, A., Tanwar, R., & Kaushik, M. (2012). Ethnomedicine: Applications of Neem (Azadirachta indica) in dentistry. Dental Hypotheses, 3(3), 112.

Prashant, G. M., Chandu, G. N., Murulikrishna, K. S., & Shafiulla, M. D. (2007). The effect of mango and neem extract on four organisms causing dental caries: Streptococcus mutans, Streptococcus salivavius, Streptococcus mitis, and Streptococcus sanguis: An in vitro study. Indian Journal of Dental Research, 18(4), 148.

Sorna, K. H., Rajasekar, T., Anandhi, A., & Shahanas, B. A. (2011). Comparative study of in vitro antibacterial activity of Neem and miswak extracts against isolated cariogens from dental caries patients. J Chem Pharm Res, 3, 638-45.

Marco, A. B., Rinaldo, A. S., Jose, G. M., Cintia, O. C., Cláudio, A. R., & Dinalva, B. Q. (2008). Efficacy of a neem mouthrinse (Azadirachta indica) in the treatment of patients with chronic gingivitis. J Med Plant Res, 2(11), 341-6.

CHAPTER - SPICES OF INDIA

Turmeric - a spice with multiple medicinal properties

Ammon, H. P., & Wahl, M. A. (1991). Pharmacology of Curcuma longa. Planta medica, 57(01), 1-7.

Araujo, C. A. C., & Leon, L. L. (2001). Biological activities of Curcuma longa L. Memórias do Instituto Oswaldo Cruz, 96(5), 723-728.

Aggarwal, B. B., Sundaram, C., Malani, N., & Ichikawa, H. (2007). Curcumin: the Indian solid gold. In The molecular targets and therapeutic uses of curcumin in health and disease (pp. 1-75). Springer, Boston, MA.

Aggarwal, B. B., & Sung, B. (2009). Pharmacological basis for the role of curcumin in chronic diseases: an age-old spice with modern targets. Trends in pharmacological sciences, 30(2), 85-94.

Zhou, H., S Beevers, C., & Huang, S. (2011). The targets of curcumin. Current drug targets, 12(3), 332-347.

Balasubramanian, K. (2006). Molecular orbital basis for yellow curry spice curcumin's prevention of Alzheimer's disease. Journal of agricultural and food chemistry, 54(10), 3512-3520.

Menon, V. P., & Sudheer, A. R. (2007). Antioxidant and anti-inflammatory properties of curcumin. In The molecular targets and therapeutic uses of curcumin in health and disease (pp. 105-125). Springer, Boston, MA.

Yanagisawa, D., Shirai, N., Amatsubo, T., Taguchi, H., Hirao, K., Urushitani, M., ... & Morino, K. (2010). Relationship between the tautomeric structures of curcumin derivatives and their Aβ-binding activities in the context of therapies for Alzheimer's disease. Biomaterials, 31(14), 4179-4185.

Yang, F., Lim, G. P., Begum, A. N., Ubeda, O. J., Simmons, M. R., Ambegaokar, S. S., ... & Cole, G. M. (2005). Curcumin inhibits formation of amyloid β oligomers and fibrils, binds plaques, and reduces amyloid in vivo. Journal of Biological Chemistry, 280(7), 5892-5901.

Lee, V. M. Y. (2002). Amyloid binding ligands as Alzheimer's disease therapies. Neurobiology of aging, 23(6), 1039-1042.

Tomiyama, T. (2010). Involvement of beta-amyloid in the etiology

of Alzheimer's disease. Brain and nerve= Shinkei kenkyu no shinpo, 62(7), 691-699.

Jurenka, J. S. (2009). Anti-inflammatory properties of curcumin, a major constituent of Curcuma longa: a review of preclinical and clinical research. Alternative medicine review, 14(2).

Jankasem, M., Wuthi-udomlert, M., & Gritsanapan, W. (2013). Antidermatophytic properties of ar-turmerone, turmeric oil, and Curcuma longa preparations. ISRN dermatology, 2013.

Kulkarni, S. J., Maske, K. N., Budre, M. P., & Mahajan, R. P. (2012). Extraction and purification of curcuminoids from Turmeric (Curcuma longa L.). International Journal of Pharmacology and Pharmaceutical Technology, 1(2), 81-84.

Chakraborty, P. S., Kausik, S., Nain, S. S., Singh, P., Singh, D., Singh, O., ... & Bawaskar, R. (2012). Staphylococcinum-A multicenter clinical verification study. Indian Journal of Research in Homoeopathy, 6(2), 15.

Kim, H. J., Yoo, H. S., Kim, J. C., Park, C. S., Choi, M. S., Kim, M., ... & Ahn, J. K. (2009). Antiviral effect of Curcuma longa Linn extract against hepatitis B virus replication. Journal of ethnopharmacology, 124(2), 189-196.

Saraf, S., Jeswani, G., Kaur, C. D., & Saraf, S. (2011). Development of novel

herbal cosmetic cream with Curcuma longa extract loaded transfersomes for antiwrinkle effect.
African journal of pharmacy and pharmacology, 5(8), 1054-1062.

Su, H. C., Horvat, R., & Jilani, G. (1982). Isolation, purification, and characterization of insect repellents from Curcuma longa L. Journal of Agricultural and Food Chemistry, 30(2), 290-292.

Salama, S. M., Abdulla, M. A., AlRashdi, A. S., Ismail, S., Alkiyumi, S. S., & Golbabapour, S. (2013). Hepatoprotective effect of ethanolic extract of Curcuma longa on thioacetamide induced liver cirrhosis in rats. BMC complementary and Alternative medicine, 13(1), 56.

Joshi, D., Mittal, D. K., Kumar, R., Kumar Srivastav, A., & Srivastav, S. K. (2013). Protective role of Curcuma longa extract and curcumin on mercuric chloride-induced nephrotoxicity

in rats: evidence by histological architecture. Toxicological & Environmental Chemistry, 95(9), 1581-1588.

Jain, R. Y. G. (2011). Effect of contragestative dose of aqueous extract of Curcuma longa rhizome on uterine biochemical milieu of female rats.

Khan, M. G., Nahar, K., Rahman, M. S., Hasan, C. M., & Rashid, M. A. (2009). Phytochemical and biological investigations of Curcuma longa. Dhaka University Journal of Pharmaceutical Sciences, 8(1), 39-45.

Cassileth, B. (2010). Turmeric (Curcuma longa, Curcuma domestica). Oncology, 24(6), 546-546.

PEPPER- Indian spice exchanged for gold

Karsha, P. V., & Lakshmi, O. B. (2010). Antibacterial activity of black pepper (Piper nigrum Linn.) with special reference to its mode of action on bacteria.

Mehmood, M. H., & Gilani, A. H. (2010). Pharmacological basis for the medicinal use of black pepper and piperine in gastrointestinal disorders. Journal of medicinal food, 13(5), 1086-1096.

Ahmad, N., Fazal, H., Abbasi, B. H., Farooq, S., Ali, M., & Khan, M. A. (2012). Biological role of Piper nigrum L.(Black pepper): A review. Asian Pacific Journal of Tropical Biomedicine, 2(3), S1945-S1953.
Nahak, G., & Sahu, R. K. (2011). Phytochemical Evaluation and Antioxidant activity of Piper cubeba and Piper nigrum.

MALABATHRUM leaves that spice your food

Chakraborty, U., & Das, H. (2010). Antidiabetic and antioxidant activities of Cinnamomum tamala leaf extracts in Stz-treated diabetic rats. Global Journal of Biotechnology & Biochemistry, 5(1), 12-18.

Kumar, S., Sharma, S., & Vasudeva, N. (2012). Chemical compositions of Cinnamomum tamala oil from two different regions of India. Asian Pacific Journal of Tropical Disease, 2, S761-S764.

Dhulasavant, V., Shinde, S., Pawar, M., & Naikwade, N. S. (2010). Antihyperlipidemic activity of Cinnamomum tamala Nees. on high cholesterol diet induced hyperlipidemia. International Journal of PharmTech Research, 2(4), 2517-2521.

Ullah, N., Khan, M. A., Khan, T., & Ahmad, W. (2013). Protective effect of Cinnamomum tamala extract on gentamicin-induced nephrotic damage in rabbits. Tropical Journal of Pharmaceutical Research, 12(2), 215-219.

Thamizhselvam, N., Soumya, S., Sanjayakumar, Y. R., Venugopalan, T. N., & Jaya, N. (2012). Anti-inflammatory, analgesic and antipyretic activity of methanolic extract of Cinnamomum tamala (nees) in experimental animal models. International Journal of Bioassays, 1(9), 26-29.
Ahmed, A., Choudhary, M. I., Farooq, A., Demirci, B., Demirci, F., & Baser,

K. C. (2000). Essential oil constituents of the spice Cinnamomum tamala (Ham.) Nees & Eberm. Flavour and Fragrance Journal, 15(6), 388-390.

Al-Mamun, R., Hamid, A., Islam, M. K., Chowdhury, J. A., & Azam, A. Z. (2011). Lipid lowering activity and free radical scavenging effect of Cinnamomum tamala (fam: Lauraceae). International Journal of Natural Sciences, 1(4), 93-96.

Kumar, S., Vasudeva, N., & Sharma, S. (2012). GC-MS analysis and screening of antidiabetic, antioxidant and hypolipidemic potential of Cinnamomum tamala oil in streptozotocin induced diabetes mellitus in rats. Cardiovascular diabetology, 11(1), 95.

CARDAMOM - the antioxidant spice

Verma, S. K., Jain, V., & Katewa, S. S. (2009). Blood pressure lowering, fibrinolysis enhancing and antioxidant activities of cardamom (Elettaria cardamomum).

A.ullah Khan, A., Khan, Q. J., & Gilani, A. H. (2011). Pharmacological basis for the medicinal use of cardamom in asthma. Bangladesh Journal of Pharmacology, 6(1), 34-37.

Kubo, I., Himejima, M., & Muroi, H. (1991). Antimicrobial activity of flavor components of cardamom Elettaria cardamomum (Zingiberaceae) seed. Journal of agricultural and food chemistry, 39(11), 1984-1986.

Padmakumari Amma, K. P. A., Venugopalan Nair, P. N., Sasidharan, I., & Priya Rani, M. (2010). Chemical composition, flavonoid-phenolic contents and radical scavenging activity of four major varieties of cardamom.

Gopalakrishnan, M. J. C. S., Narayanan, C. S., & Grenz, M. (1990). Nonsaponifiable lipid constituents of Cardamom. Journal of agricultural and food chemistry, 38(12), 2133-2136.

Kaushik, P., Goyal, P., Chauhan, A., & Chauhan, G. (2010). In vitro evaluation of antibacterial potential of dry fruitextracts of Elettaria cardamomum Maton (Chhoti Elaichi). Iranian journal of pharmaceutical research: IJPR, 9(3), 287.

El Malti, J., Mountassif, D., & Amarouch, H. (2007). Antimicrobial activity of Elettaria cardamomum: Toxicity, biochemical and histological studies. Food chemistry, 104(4), 1560-1568.

Jamal, A., Javed, K., Aslam, M., & Jafri, M. A. (2006). Gastroprotective effect of cardamom, Elettaria cardamomum Maton. fruits in rats. Journal of ethnopharmacology, 103(2), 149-153.

Gilani, A. H., Jabeen, Q., Khan, A. U., & Shah, A. J. (2008). Gut modulatory, blood pressure lowering, diuretic and sedative activities of cardamom. Journal of ethnopharmacology, 115(3), 463-472.

Al-Zuhair, H., El-Sayeh, B., Ameen, H. A., & Al-Shoora, H. (1996). Pharmacological studies of cardamom oil in animals. Pharmacological research, 34(1-2), 79-82.

Badei, A. Z. M., Morsi, H. H. H., & El-Akel, A. T. M. (1991). Chemical composition and antioxidant properties of cardamom essential oil. Bulletin of Faculty of Agriculture, Cairo Univ.(Egypt).

Huang, Y., Lam, S. L., & Ho, S. H. (2000). Bioactivities of essential oil from Elletaria cardamomum (L.) Maton. to Sitophilus zeamais Motschulsky and: Tribolium castaneum (Herbst). Journal of Stored Products Research, 36(2), 107-117.

Suneetha, W. J., & Krishnakantha, T. P. (2005). Cardamom extract as inhibitor of human platelet aggregation. Phytotherapy Research, 19(5), 437-440.

Achliya, G. S., Wadodkar, S. G., & Dorle, A. K. (2004). Evaluation of sedative and anticonvulsant activities of Unmadnashak Ghrita. Journal of ethnopharmacology, 94(1), 77-83.

Balaji, S., & Chempakam, B. (2008). Mutagenicity and carcinogenicity prediction of compounds from cardamom (Elettaria cardamom Maton). Ethnobotanical Leaflets, 2008(1), 91.

Verma, S. K., Rajeevan, V., Bordia, A., & Jain, V. (2010). Greater cardamom (Amomum subulatum Roxb.)–A cardio-adaptogen against physical stress. J. Herb. Med. Toxicol, 4(2), 55-58.

Verma, S. K., Jain, V., & Singh, D. P. (2012). Effect of Greater cardamom (Amomum subulatum Roxb.) on blood lipids, fibrinolysis and total antioxidant status in patients with ischemic heart disease. Asian Pacific Journal of Tropical Disease, 2, S739-S743.

Bisht, V. K., Negi, J. S., Bh, A. K., & Sundriyal, R. C. (2011). Amomum subulatum Roxb: Traditional, phytochemical and biological activities-An overview. African Journal of Agricultural Research, 6(24), 5386-5390.

Lakshmi, V. (1977). Structure of a new aurone glycoside from Amomum subulatum seeds. Indian J Chem Sect B, 15, 814-815.

Agnihotri, S. A., Wakode, S. R., & Ali, M. (2012). Chemical composition, antimicrobial and topical anti-inflammatory activity of essential oil of Amomum subulatum fruits. Acta Poloniae Pharmaceutican Drug Res, 69(6), 1177-81.

Shukla, S. H., Mistry, H. A., Patel, V. G., & Jogi, B. V. (2010). Pharmacognostical, preliminary phytochemical studies and analgesic activity of Amomum subulatum Roxb. Pharma Science Monitor, 1(1), 90-102.

Alam, K., Pathak, D., & Ansari, S. H. (2011). Evaluation of anti-inflammatory activity of Ammomum subulatum fruit extract. Int. J. Pharmaceu. Sci. Drug. Res, 3(1), 35-37.

Kumar, U., Kumar, B., Bhandari, A., & Kumar, Y. (2010). Phytochemical investigation and comparison of antimicrobial screening of clove and cardamom. Int J Pharm Sci Res, 1, 138-147.

Jain, P. C., & Agarwal, S. C. (1976). Activity of some plants extracts against some keratinophilic species of Nannizzia. Ind. Drugs, 23(12), 25-26.

Hussain, T., Arshad, M., Khan, S., Sattar, H., & Qureshi, M. S. (2011). In vitro screening of methanol plant extracts for their antibacterial activity. Pak J Bot, 43(1), 531-538.

Aneja, K. R., & Joshi, R. (2009). Antimicrobial activity of Amomum subulatum and Elettaria cardamomum against dental caries causing microorganisms. Ethnobotanical Leaflets, 2009(7), 3.

Kikuzaki, H., Kawai, Y., & Nakatani, N. (2001). 1, 1-Diphenyl-2-picrylhydrazyl radical-scavenging active compounds from greater cardamom (Amomum subulatum Roxb.). Journal of nutritional science and vitaminology, 47(2), 167-171.

Verma, S. K., Rajeevan, V., Bordia, A., & Jain, V. (2010). Greater cardamom (Amomum subulatum Roxb.)–A cardio-adaptogen against physical stress. J. Herb. Med. Toxicol, 4(2), 55-58.

Jafri, M. A., Javed, K., & Singh, S. (2001). Evaluation of the gastric antiulcerogenic effect of large cardamom (fruits of Amomum subulatum Roxb). Journal of Ethnopharmacology, 75(2-3), 89-94.

Jamal, A., Siddiqui, A., Aslam, M., Javed, K., & Jafri, M. A. (2005). Antiulcerogenic activity of Elettaria cardamomum Maton. and Amomum subulatum Roxb. seeds.

Parmar, M., Shah, P., Thakkar, V., & Gandhi, T. (2009). Hepatoprotective activity of Amomum subulatum Roxb against ethanol-induced liver damage.

International Journal of Green Pharmacy, 3(3), 250.

Vavaiya, R. B., Patel, A., & Manek, R. A. (2010). Anti-diabetic activity of Amomum subulatum Roxb. fruit constituents. IJPI, 2(5), 50-63.
Dhuley, J. N. (1999). Anti-oxidant effects of cinnamon (Cinnamomum verum) bark and greater cardamom (Amomum subulatum) seeds in rats fed high fat diet.

CHAPTER CHINESE HERBS

Ni, M. (1995). The Yellow Emperor's classic of medicine: a new translation of the Neijing Suwen with commentary. Shambhala Publications.

GARLIC and its myriad medicinal properties

Petrovska, B. B., & Cekovska, S. (2010). Extracts from the history and medical properties of garlic. Pharmacognosy reviews, 4(7), 106.

Ackermann, R. T., Mulrow, C. D., Ramirez, G., Gardner, C. D., Morbidoni, L., & Lawrence, V. A. (2001). Garlic shows promise for improving some cardiovascular risk factors. Archives of internal medicine, 161(6), 813-824.

Berthold, H. K., & Sudhop, T. (1998). Garlic preparations for prevention of atherosclerosis. Current opinion in lipidology, 9(6), 565-569.

Ashraf, R., Aamir, K., Shaikh, A. R., & Ahmed, T. (2005). Effects of garlic on dyslipidemia in patients with type 2 diabetes mellitus. J Ayub Med Coll Abbottabad, 17(3), 60-64.

Borrelli, F., Capasso, R., & Izzo, A. A. (2007). Garlic (Allium sativum L.): adverse effects and drug interactions in humans. Molecular nutrition & food research, 51(11), 1386-1397.

Dillon, S. A., Burmi, R. S., Lowe, G. M., Billington, D., & Rahman, K. (2003).

Antioxidant properties of aged garlic extract: an in vitro study incorporating human low density lipoprotein. Life sciences, 72(14), 1583-1594.

Dorant, E., van den Brandt, P. A., & Goldbohm, R. A. (1996). A prospective cohort study on the relationship between onion and leek consumption, garlic supplement use and the risk of colorectal carcinoma in The Netherlands. Carcinogenesis, 17(3), 477-484.

Yılmaz, E., Devrim, E., Perk, H., & Kaçmaz, M. (2003). Consumption of aqueous garlic extract leads to significant improvement in patients with benign prostate hyperplasia and prostate cancer. Nutrition research, 23(2), 199-204.

Fleischauer, A. T., Poole, C., & Arab, L. (2000). Garlic consumption and cancer prevention: meta-analyses of colorectal and stomach cancers–. The American journal of clinical nutrition, 72(4), 1047-1052.

Fugh-Berman, A. (2000). Herbs and dietary supplements in the prevention and treatment of cardiovascular disease. Preventive Cardiology, 3(1), 24-32.

Sussman, E. (2002). Garlic supplements can impede HIV medication. AIDS (London, England), 16(9), N5.

Gallicano, K., Foster, B., & Choudhri, S. (2003). Effect of short-term administration of garlic supplements on single-dose ritonavir pharmacokinetics in healthy volunteers. British journal of clinical pharmacology, 55(2), 199-202.

Gullett, N. P., Amin, A. R., Bayraktar, S., Pezzuto, J. M., Shin, D. M., Khuri, F. R., ... & Kucuk, O. (2010, June). Cancer prevention with natural compounds. In Seminars in oncology(Vol. 37, No. 3, pp.258-281). Elsevier.

Heron, S., & Yarnell, E. (1999). Treating parasitic infections with botanical medicines. Alternative and Complementary Therapies, 5(4), 214-224.

Isaacsohn, J. L., Moser, M., Stein, E. A., Dudley, K., Davey, J. A., Liskov,

E., & Black, H. R. (1998). Garlic powder and plasma lipids and lipoproteins: a multicenter, randomized, placebo-controlled trial. Archives of Internal Medicine, 158(11), 1189-1194.

Izzo, A. A., & Ernst, E. (2001). Interactions between herbal medicines and prescribed drugs. Drugs, 61(15), 2163-2175.

James, J. S. (2001). Garlic reduces saquinavir blood levels 50%; may affect other drugs. AIDS treatment news, (375), 2-3.

Ngo, S. N., Williams, D. B., Cobiac, L., & Head, R. J. (2007). Does garlic reduce risk of colorectal cancer? A systematic review. The Journal of nutrition, 137(10), 2264-2269.

Nies, L. K., Cymbala, A. A., Kasten, S. L., Lamprecht, D. G., & Olson, K. L. (2006). Complementary and alternative therapies for the management of dyslipidemia. Annals of Pharmacotherapy, 40(11), 1984-1992.

O'Gara, E. A., Maslin, D. J., Nevill, A. M., & Hill, D. J. (2008). The effect of simulated gastric environments on the anti-Helicobacter activity of garlic oil. Journal of applied microbiology, 104(5), 1324-1331.

Ried, K., Frank, O. R., & Stocks, N. P. (2010). Aged garlic extract lowers blood pressure in patients with treated but uncontrolled hypertension: a randomised controlled trial. Maturitas, 67(2), 144-150.

Sarrell, E. M., Mandelberg, A., & Cohen, H. A. (2001). Efficacy of naturopathic extracts in the management of ear pain associated with acute otitis media. Archives of pediatrics & adolescent medicine, 155(7), 796-799.

Salih, B. A., & Abasiyanik, F. M. (2003). Does regular garlic intake affect the prevalence of Helicobacter pylori in asymptomatic subjects?. Saudi medical journal, 24(8), 842-845.

Sobenin, I. A., Pryanishnikov, V. V., Kunnova, L. M., Rabinovich, Y. A.,

Martirosyan, D. M., & Orekhov, A. N. (2010). The effects of time-released garlic powder tablets on multifunctional cardiovascular risk in patients with coronary artery disease. Lipids in health and disease, 9(1), 119.

Stevinson, C., Pittler, M. H., & Ernst, E. (2000). Garlic for treating hypercholesterolemia: a meta-analysis of randomized clinical trials. Annals of internal medicine, 133(6), 420-429.

Superko, H. R., & Krauss, R. M. (2000). Garlic powder, effect on plasma lipids, postprandial lipemia, low-density lipoprotein particle size, high-density lipoprotein subclass distribution and lipoprotein (a). Journal of the American College of Cardiology, 35(2), 321-326.

Wang, H. X., & Ng, T. B. (1999). Natural products with hypoglycemic, hypotensive, hypocholesterolemic, antiatherosclerotic and antithrombotic activities. Life sciences, 65(25), 2663-2677.

Block, E. (1992). The organosulfur chemistry of the genus Allium– implications for the organic chemistry of sulfur. Angewandte Chemie International Edition in English, 31(9), 1135-1178. '

IDE, N., & LAU, B. H. (1997). Garlic compounds protect vascular endothelial cells from oxidized low density lipoprotein-induced injury. Journal of pharmacy and pharmacology, 49(9), 908-911.

Koch, H. P., & Lawson, L. D. (1996). Garlic: the science and therapeutic application of Allium sativum L. and related species (Vol. 683181475). baltimore, Maryland: Williams & Wilkins xv, 329p. ISBN.

Moyers, S. B. (1996). Garlic in health, history, and world cuisine (Vol. 3, pp. 1-36). St. Petersburg, FL: Suncoast Press.

Riddle, J. M. (1996). The medicines of Greco-Roman antiquity as a source of medicines for today. Prospecting for Drugs in Ancient and Medieval European Texts: A Scientific Approach, 7-17.

Steiner, M., & Lin, R. S. (1998). Changes in platelet function and susceptibility of lipoproteins to oxidation associated with administration of aged garlic extract. Journal of cardiovascular pharmacology, 31(6), 904-908.

ONION not just vegetable but also medicine

Azu, N. C., & Onyeagba, R. A. (2007). Antimicrobial properties of extracts of Allium cepa (Onions) and Zingiber officinale (Ginger) on Escherichia coli, Salmonella typhi, and Bacillus subtilis. The internet journal of tropical medicine, 3(2), 8.

Votto, A. P., Domingues, B. S., de Souza, M. M., da Silva Júnior, F. M., Caldas, S. S., Filgueira, D., … & Trindade, G. S. (2010). Toxicity mechanisms of onion (Allium cepa) extracts and compounds in multidrug resistant erythroleukemic cell line. Biological research, 43(4), 429-437.

Draelos, Z. D., Baumann, L., & Fleischer, A. B. (2012). A new proprietary onion extract gel improves the appearance of new scars: a randomized, controlled, blinded-investigator study. The Journal of clinical and aesthetic dermatology, 5(6), 18.

GINGER and their little known medicinal properties

Altman, R. D., & Marcussen, K. C. (2001). Effects of a ginger extract on knee pain in patients with osteoarthritis. Arthritis & Rheumatology, 44(11), 2531-2538.

Wigler, I., Grotto, I., Caspi, D., & Yaron, M. (2003). The effects of Zintona EC (a ginger extract) on symptomatic gonarthritis. Osteoarthritis and cartilage, 11(11), 783-789.

Apariman, S., Ratchanon, S., & Wiriyasirivej, B. (2006). Effectiveness of ginger for prevention of nausea and vomiting after gynecological laparoscopy. Journal-Medical Association of Thailand, 89(12), 2003.

Ali, B. H., Blunden, G., Tanira, M. O., & Nemmar, A. (2008). Some phytochemical, pharmacological and toxicological properties of ginger (Zingiber officinale Roscoe): a review of recent research. Food and chemical Toxicology, 46(2), 409-420.

Bone, M. E., Wilkinson, D. J., Young, J. R., McNeil, J., & Charlton, S. (1990). Ginger root—a new antiemetic The effect of ginger root on postoperative nausea and vomiting after major gynaecological surgery. Anaesthesia, 45(8), 669-671.

Chaiyakunapruk, N., Kitikannakorn, N., Nathisuwan, S., Leeprakobboon, K., & Leelasettagool, C. (2006). The efficacy of ginger for the prevention of postoperative nausea and vomiting: a meta-analysis. American Journal of Obstetrics & Gynecology, 194(1), 95-99.

Eberhart, L. H., Mayer, R., Betz, O., Tsolakidis, S., Hilpert, W., Morin, A. M., ... & Seeling, W. (2003). Ginger does not prevent postoperative nausea and vomiting after laparoscopic surgery. Anesthesia & Analgesia, 96(4), 995-998.

Kalava, A., Darji, S. J., Kalstein, A., Yarmush, J. M., SchianodiCola, J., & Weinberg, J. (2013). Efficacy of ginger on intraoperative and postoperative nausea and vomiting in elective cesarean section patients. European Journal of Obstetrics and Gynecology and Reproductive Biology, 169(2), 184-188.

Langner, E., Greifenberg, S., & Gruenwald, J. (1998). Ginger: history and use. Advances in therapy, 15(1), 25-44.

Larkin, M. (1999). Surgery patients at risk for herb-anaesthesia interactions. The Lancet, 354(9187), 1362.

Phillips, S., Ruggier, R., & Hutchinson, S. E. (1993). Zingiber officinale (ginger)–an antiemetic for day case surgery. Anaesthesia, 48(8), 715-717.

Pongrojpaw, D., Somprasit, C., & Chanthasenanont, A. (2007). A randomized comparison of ginger and dimenhydrinate in the treatment of nausea and vomiting in pregnancy. Journal-Medical Association of Thailand, 90(9), 1703.

Portnoi, G., Chng, L. A., Karimi-Tabesh, L., Koren, G., Tan, M. P., & Einarson, A. (2003). Prospective comparative study of the safety and effectiveness of ginger for the treatment of nausea and vomiting in pregnancy. American Journal of Obstetrics & Gynecology, 189(5), 1374-1377.

Sripramote, M., & Lekhyananda, N. (2003). A randomized comparison of ginger and vitamin B6 in the treatment of nausea and vomiting of pregnancy. Journal of the Medical Association of Thailand Chotmaihet thangphaet, 86(9), 846-853.

Viljoen, E., Visser, J., Koen, N., & Musekiwa, A. (2014). A systematic review and meta-analysis of the effect and safety of ginger in the treatment of pregnancy-associated nausea and vomiting. Nutrition journal, 13(1), 20.

Vutyavanich, T., Kraisarin, T., & Ruangsri, R. A. (2001). Ginger for nausea and vomiting in pregnancy:: Randomized, double-masked, placebo-controlled trial. Obstetrics & Gynecology, 97(4), 577-582.

Willetts, K. E., Ekangaki, A., & Eden, J. A. (2003). Effect of a ginger extract on pregnancy-induced nausea: A randomised controlled trial. Australian and New Zealand journal of obstetrics and gynaecology, 43(2), 139-144.

Grøntved, A., Brask, T., Kambskard, J., & Hentzer, E. (1988). Ginger Root Against Seasickness: A Conctrolled Trial on the Open Sea. Acta oto-laryngologica, 105(1-2), 45-49.

Gregory, P. J., Sperry, M., & Wilson, A. F. (2008). Dietary supplements for osteoarthritis. American family physician, 77(2).

Bordia, A., Verma, S. K., & Srivastava, K. C. (1997). Effect of ginger (Zingiber officinale Rosc.) and fenugreek (Trigonella foenumgraecum L.) on blood lipids, blood sugar and platelet aggregation in patients with coronary artery disease. Prostaglandins, Leukotrienes and Essential Fatty Acids, 56(5), 379-384.

Fuhrman, B., Rosenblat, M., Hayek, T., Coleman, R., & Aviram, M. (2000). Ginger extract consumption reduces plasma cholesterol, inhibits LDL oxidation and attenuates development of atherosclerosis in atherosclerotic, apolipoprotein E-deficient mice. The Journal of nutrition, 130(5), 1124-1131.

Nurtjahja-Tjendraputra, E., Ammit, A. J., Roufogalis, B. D., Tran, V. H., & Duke, C. C. (2003). Effective anti-platelet and COX-1 enzyme inhibitors from pungent constituents of ginger. Thrombosis research, 111(4), 259-265.

Thomson, M., Al-Qattan, K. K., Al-Sawan, S. M., Alnaqeeb, M. A.,Khan, I., & Ali, M. (2002). The use of ginger (Zingiber officinale Rosc.) as a potential anti-inflammatory and antithrombotic agent. Prostaglandins, leukotrienes and essential fatty acids, 67(6), 475-478.

Lee, S. H., Cekanova, M., & Baek, S. J. (2008). Multiple mechanisms are involved in 6-gingerol-induced cell growth arrest and apoptosis in human colorectal cancer cells. Molecular carcinogenesis, 47(3), 197-208.

Wang, C. C., Chen, L. G., Lee, L. T., & Yang, L. L. (2003). Effects of 6-gingerol, an antioxidant from ginger, on inducing apoptosis in human leukemic HL-60 cells. In vivo (Athens, Greece), 17(6), 641-645.

Mahady, G. B., Pendland, S. L., Yun, G. S., Lu, Z. Z., & Stoia, A. (2003). Ginger (Zingiber officinale Roscoe) and the gingerols inhibit the growth of Cag A+ strains of Helicobacter pylori. Anticancer research, 23, 3699.

Vaes, L. P., & Chyka, P. A. (2000). Interactions of warfarin with garlic, ginger, ginkgo, or ginseng: nature of the evidence. Annals of Pharmacotherapy, 34(12), 1478-1482.

Fischer-Rasmussen, W., Kjær, S. K., Dahl, C., & Asping, U. (1991). Ginger treatment of hyperemesis gravidarum. European Journal of Obstetrics &

Gynecology, 38(1), 19-24.

Star anise a cure for bird flu

Orwa, C., Mutua, A., Kindt, R., Jamnadass, R., & Simons, A. (2009). Agroforestree database: a tree species reference and selection guide version 4.0. World Agroforestry Centre ICRAF, Nairobi, KE.

Chang, K. S., & Ahn, Y. J. (2002). Fumigant activity of (E)-anethole identified in Illicium verum fruit against Blattella germanica. Pest management science, 58(2), 161-166.

De, M., De, A. K., Sen, P., & Banerjee, A. B. (2002). Antimicrobial properties of star anise (Illicium verum Hook f). Phytotherapy Research, 16(1), 94-95.

Garzo, C. F., Gómez, P. P., Barrasa, A. B., Martínez, R. A., Ramírez, R. F., & Ramón, F. R. (2002). Cases of neurological symptoms associated with star anise consumption used as a carminative. Anales espanoles de pediatria, 57(4), 290-294.

Ize-Ludlow, D., Ragone, S., Bruck, I. S., Bernstein, J. N., Duchowny, M., & Peña, B. M. G. (2004). Neurotoxicities in infants seen with the consumption of star anise tea. Pediatrics, 114(5), e653-e656.

Ghosh, S., Chisti, Y., & Banerjee, U. C. (2012). Production of shikimic acid. Biotechnology advances, 30(6), 1425-1431.

Sichuan pepper a culinary spice that tingles and numbs at the same time

Austin, D. F., & Felger, R. S. (2008). Sichuan peppers and the etymology of fagara (Rutaceae). Economic botany, 62(4), 567-573.

Prempeh, A. B. A. (2008). Analgesic activity of crude aqueous extract of the root bark of Zanthoxylum Xanthoxyloides. Ghana medical journal, 42(2).

Lima, L. M., Perazzo, F. F., Carvalho, J. C. T., & Bastos, J. K. (2007). Anti-inflammatory and analgesic activities of the ethanolic extracts from Zanthoxylum riedelianum (Rutaceae) leaves and stem bark. Journal of Pharmacy and Pharmacology, 59(8), 1151-1158.

Chen, J. J., Lin, Y. H., Day, S. H., Hwang, T. L., & Chen, I. S. (2011). New benzenoids and anti-inflammatory constituents from Zanthoxylum nitidum. Food chemistry, 125(2), 282-287.

Wan, H. C., Hu, D. Y., & Liu, H. C. (2005). Clinical observation of toothpaste containing Zanthoxylum nitidum extract on dental plaque and gingivitis. Zhongguo Zhong xi yi jie he za zhi Zhongguo Zhongxiyi jiehe zazhi= Chinese journal of integrated traditional and Western medicine, 25(11), 1024-1026.

Guo, T., Deng, Y. X., Xie, H., Yao, C. Y., Cai, C. C., Pan, S. L., & Wang, Y. L. (2011). Antinociceptive and anti-inflammatory activities of ethyl acetate fraction from Zanthoxylum armatum in mice. Fitoterapia, 82(3), 347-351.

Dongmo, P. M. J., Tchoumbougnang, F., Sonwa, E. T., Kenfack, S. M., Zollo, P. H. A., & Menut, C. (2008). Antioxidant and antiinflammatory potential of essential oils of some Zanthoxylum (Rutaceae) of Cameroon. International journal of essential oil therapeutics, 2(2), 82-88.

Manandhar, A., & Tiwari, R. D. (2005). Antifungal efficacy of Zanthoxylum oil against Bipolaris sorokiniana (Sacc.)

Shoem. Ecoprint: An International Journal of Ecology, 12, 91-93.

Bafi-Yeboa, N. F. A., Arnason, J. T., Baker, J., & Smith, M. L. (2005). Antifungal constituents of Northern prickly ash, Zanthoxylum americanum Mill. Phytomedicine, 12(5), 370-377.

Mehta, D. K., Das, R., & Bhandari, A. (2012). In-vitro anthelmintic activity of seeds of Zanthoxylum armatum DC. against Pheretima Posthuma. International Journal of Green Pharmacy (IJGP), 6(1).

Zirihi, G. N., N'guessan, K., Etien, D. T., & Seri-Kouassi, B. (2009). Evaluation in vitro of antiplasmodial activity of ethanolic extracts of Funtumia elastica, Rauvolfia vomitoria and Zanthoxylum gilletii on Plasmodium falciparum isolates from Côte-d'Ivoire. Journal of Animal and Plant Sciences (JAPS), 5(1), 406-413.

Batool, F. A. R. H. A. T., Sabir, S. M., Rocha, J. B. T., Shah, A. H., Saify, Z. S., & Ahmed, S. D. (2010). Evaluation of antioxidant and free radical scavenging activities of fruit extract from Zanthoxylum alatum: a commonly used spice from Pakistan. Pak J Bot, 42(6), 4299-311.

Hisatomi, E., Matsui, M., Kubota, K., & Kobayashi, A. (2000). Antioxidative activity in the pericarp and seed of Japanese pepper (Xanthoxylum piperitum DC). Journal of agricultural and food chemistry, 48(10), 4924-4928.

Xia, L., You, J., Li, G., Sun, Z., & Suo, Y. (2011). Compositional and antioxidant activity analysis of Zanthoxylum bungeanum seed oil obtained by supercritical CO_2 fluid extraction. Journal of the American Oil Chemists' Society, 88(1), 23-32.

Yamazaki, E., Inagaki, M., Kurita, O., & Inoue, T. (2007). Antioxidant activity of Japanese pepper (Zanthoxylum piperitum DC.) fruit. Food chemistry, 100(1), 171-177.

Amabeoku, G. J., & Kinyua, C. G. (2010). Evaluation of the anticonvulsant activity of Zanthoxylum capense (Thunb.) Harv. (Rutaceae) in mice.

Gilani, S. N., Khan, A. U., & Gilani, A. H. (2010). Pharmacological basis for the medicinal use of Zanthoxylum armatum in gut, airways and cardiovascular disorders. Phytotherapy research, 24(4), 553-558.

Lee, S. J., & Lim, K. T. (2008). Glycoprotein of Zanthoxylum piperitum DC has a hepatoprotective effect via anti-oxidative character in vivo and in vitro. Toxicology in vitro, 22(2), 376-385.

Suryanto, E., Sastrohamidjojo, H., & Raharjo, S. (2004). Antiradical Activity of Andaliman (Zanthoxylumachanthopodium DC) Fruit Extract. Indonesian Food and Nutrition Progress, 11(1), 15-19.

Jullian, V., Bourdy, G., Georges, S., Maurel, S., & Sauvain, M. (2006). Validation of use of a traditional antimalarial remedy from French Guiana, Zanthoxylum rhoifolium Lam. Journal of Ethnopharmacology, 106(3), 348-352.

Fennel an aftermeal digestive

Oktay, M., Gülçin, İ., & Küfrevioğlu, Ö. İ. (2003). Determination of in vitro antioxidant activity of fennel (Foeniculum vulgare) seed extracts. LWT-Food Science and Technology, 36(2), 263-271.

Anwar, F., Ali, M., Hussain, A. I., & Shahid, M. (2009). Antioxidant and antimicrobial activities of essential oil and extracts of fennel (Foeniculum vulgare Mill.) seeds from Pakistan. Flavour and Fragrance Journal, 24(4), 170-176.

Kaur, G. J., & Arora, D. S. (2009). Antibacterial and phytochemical screening of Anethum graveolens, Foeniculum vulgare and Trachyspermum ammi. BMC complementary and alternative medicine, 9(1), 30.

Manonmani, R., & Khadir, V. A. (2011). Antibacterial screening on Foeniculum vulgare Mill. International Journal of Pharma and Bio Sciences, 2(4), 390-394.

Esquivel-Ferriño, P. C., Favela-Hernández, J. M. J., Garza-González, E., Waksman, N., Ríos, M. Y., & Camacho-Corona, M. D. R. (2012). Antimycobacterial activity of constituents from Foeniculum vulgare var. dulce grown in Mexico. Molecules, 17(7), 8471-8482.

MALINI, T., Vanithakumari, G., DEVI, N. M. S. A. K., & FIANGO, V. (1985). EFFECT OF FOENICULUAI VULGARE. MILL SEED EXTRACT ON THE GENITAL ORGANS OF MALE AND FEMALE RATS.

El-Soud, N., El-Laithy, N., El-Saeed, G., Wahby, M., Khalil, M., Morsy, F., & Shaffie, N. (2011). Antidiabetic activities of Foeniculum vulgare mill. Essential oil in streptozotocin-induced diabetic rats. Macedonian Journal of Medical Sciences, 4(2), 139-146.

Koppula, S., & Kumar, H. (2013). Foeniculum vulgare Mill (Umbelliferae) attenuates stress and improves memory in wister rats. Tropical Journal of Pharmaceutical Research, 12(4), 553-558.

Ostad, S. N., Soodi, M., Shariffzadeh, M., Khorshidi, N., & Marzban, H. (2001). The effect of fennel essential oil on uterine contraction as a model for dysmenorrhea, pharmacology and toxicology study. Journal of Ethnopharmacology, 76(3), 299-304.

Özbek, H., Uğraş, S., Dülger, H., Bayram, I., Tuncer, I., Öztürk, G., & Öztürk, A. (2003). Hepatoprotective effect of Foeniculum vulgare essential oil. Fitoterapia, 74(3), 317-319.

Pradhan, M., Sribhuwaneswari, S., Karthikeyan, D., Minz, S., Sure, P., Chandu, A. N., ... & Sivakumar, T. (2008). In-vitro cytoprotection activity of Foeniculum vulgare and Helicteres isora in cultured human blood lymphocytes and antitumour activity against B16F10 melanoma cell line. Research Journal of Pharmacy and Technology, 1(4), 450-452.

Park, S. H., & Seong, I. (2010). Antifungal effects of the extracts and essential oils from Foeniculum vulgare and Illicium verum against Candida albicans.

Korean Journal of Medical Mycology, 15(4), 157-164.

Thakur, N., Sareen, N., Shama, B., & Jagota, K. (2013). Studies on in vitro antifungal activity of Foeniculum vulgare Mill. against spoilage fungi. Global Journal of Bio-Science and BioTechnology, 2(3), 427-430.

Badgujar, S. B., Patel, V. V., & Bandivdekar, A. H. (2014). Foeniculum vulgare Mill: a review of its botany, phytochemistry, pharmacology, contemporary application, and toxicology. BioMed research international, 2014.

Lee, H. S. (2004). Acaricidal activity of constituents identified in Foeniculum vulgare fruit oil against Dermatophagoides spp.(Acari: Pyroglyphidae). Journal of agricultural and food chemistry, 52(10), 2887-2889.

Sedaghat, M. M., Dehkordi, A. S., Abai, M. R., Khanavi, M., Mohtarami, F., Abadi, Y. S., ... & Vatandoost, H. A. S. S. A. N. (2011). Larvicidal activity of essential oils of Apiaceae plants against malaria vector, Anopheles stephensi. Iranian journal of arthropod-borne diseases, 5(2), 51.

Rahimi, R., & Ardekani, M. R. S. (2013). Medicinal properties of Foeniculum vulgare Mill. in traditional Iranian medicine and modern phytotherapy. Chinese journal of integrative medicine, 19(1), 73-79.

Ghanem, M. T., Radwan, H. M., Mahdy, E. S. M., Elkholy, Y. M., Hassanein, H. D., & Shahat, A. A. (2012). Phenolic compounds from Foeniculum vulgare (Subsp. Piperitum)(Apiaceae) herb and evaluation of hepatoprotective antioxidant activity. Pharmacognosy research, 4(2), 104.

Oulmouden, F., Saïle, R., Gnaoui, N. E., Benomar, H., Lkhider, M., Amrani, S., & Ghalim, N. (2011). Hypolipidemic and anti-atherogenic effect of aqueous extract of fennel (Foeniculum Vulgare) extract in an experimental model of atherosclerosis induced by triton WR-1339. European Journal of Scientific Research, 52(1), 91-99.

De Marino, S., Gala, F., Borbone, N., Zollo, F., Vitalini, S., Visioli, F., &

Iorizzi, M. (2007). Phenolic glycosides from Foeniculum vulgare fruit and evaluation of antioxidative activity. Phytochemistry, 68(13), 1805-1812.

Tognolini, M., Ballabeni, V., Bertoni, S., Bruni, R., Impicciatore, M., & Barocelli, E. (2007). Protective effect of Foeniculum vulgare essential oil and anethole in an experimental model of thrombosis. Pharmacological research, 56(3), 254-260.

Abdul-Ghani, A. S., & Amin, R. (1988). The vascular action of aqueous extracts of Foeniculum vulgare leaves. Journal of ethnopharmacology, 24(2-3), 213-218.

Bardai, S. E., Lyoussi, B., Wibo, M., & Morel, N. (2001). Pharmacological evidence of hypotensive activity of Marrubium vulgare and Foeniculum vulgare in spontaneously hypertensive rat. Clinical and experimental hypertension, 23(4), 329-343.

Rasul, A., Akhtar, N., Khan, B. A., Mahmood, T., Zaman, S. U., & Khan, H. M. (2012). Formulation development of a cream containing fennel extract: in vivo evaluation for anti-aging effects. Die Pharmazie-An International Journal of Pharmaceutical Sciences, 67(1), 54-58.

Choi, E. M., & Hwang, J. K. (2004). Antiinflammatory, analgesic and antioxidant activities of the fruit of Foeniculum vulgare. Fitoterapia, 75(6), 557-565.

Kishore, R. N., Anjaneyulu, N., Ganesh, M. N., & Sravya, N. (2012). Evaluation of anxiolytic activity of ethanolic extract of Foeniculum vulgare in mice model. Int J Pharm Pharm Sci, 4(3), 584-586.

Joshi, H., & Parle, M. (2006). Cholinergic basis of memory-strengthening effect of Foeniculum vulgare Linn. Journal of medicinal food, 9(3), 413-417.

Mohamad, R. H., El-Bastawesy, A. M., Abdel-Monem, M. G., Noor, A. M., Al-Mehdar, H. A. R., Sharawy, S. M., & El-Merzabani, M. M. (2011).

Antioxidant and anticarcinogenic effects of methanolic extract and volatile oil of fennel seeds (Foeniculum vulgare). Journal of medicinal food, 14(9), 986-1001.

Agarwal, R. E. N. U., Gupta, S. K., Agrawal, S. S., Srivastava, S., & Saxena, R. O. H. I. T. (2008). Oculohypotensive effects of Foeniculum vulgare in experimental models of glaucoma. Indian J. Physiol. Pharmacol, 52(1), 77-83.

Bogucka-Kocka, A., Smolarz, H. D., & Kocki, J. (2008). Apoptotic activities of ethanol extracts from some Apiaceae on human leukaemia cell lines. Fitoterapia, 79(7-8), 487-497.

Tripathi, P., Tripathi, R., Patel, R. K., & Pancholi, S. S. (2013). Investigation of antimutagenic potential of Foeniculum vulgare essential oil on cyclophosphamide induced genotoxicity and oxidative stress in mice. Drug and chemical toxicology, 36(1), 35-41.

Al-Harbi, M. M., Qureshi, S., Raza, M., Ahmed, M. M., Giangreco, A. B., & Shah, A. H. (1995). Influence of anethole treatment on the tumour induced by Ehrlich ascites carcinoma cells in paw of Swiss albino mice. European journal of cancer prevention: the official journal of the European Cancer Prevention Organisation (ECP), 4(4), 307-318.

CLOVE- an antioxidant more powerful than blueberry

Lane, B. W., Ellenhorn, M. J., Hulbert, T. V., & McCarron, M. (1991). Clove oil ingestion in an infant. Human & experimental toxicology, 10(4), 291-294.

Yoo, C. B., Han, K. T., Cho, K. S., Ha, J., Park, H. J., Nam, J. H., …
& Lee, K. T. (2005). Eugenol isolated from the essential oil of Eugenia caryophyllata induces a reactive oxygen species-mediated apoptosis in HL-60 human promyelocytic leukemia cells. Cancer Letters, 225(1), 41-52.

Raghavenra, H., Diwakr, B. T., Lokesh, B. R., & Naidu, K. A. (2006).

Eugenol—The active principle from cloves inhibits 5-lipoxygenase activity and leukotriene-C4 in human PMNL cells. Prostaglandins, leukotrienes and essential fatty acids, 74(1), 23-27.

Thompson, D. C., Constantin-Teodosiu, D., & Moldéus, P. (1991). Metabolism and cytotoxicity of eugenol in isolated rat hepatocytes. Chemico-biological interactions, 77(2), 137-147.

Li, Y., Xu, C., Zhang, Q., Liu, J. Y., & Tan, R. X. (2005). In vitro anti-Helicobacter pylori action of 30 Chinese herbal medicines used to treat ulcer diseases. Journal of ethnopharmacology, 98(3), 329-333.

Smith-Palmer, A., Stewart, J., & Fyfe, L. (2004). Influence of subinhibitory concentrations of plant essential oils on the production of enterotoxins A and B and α-toxin by Staphylococcus aureus. Journal of medical microbiology, 53(10), 1023-1027.

Bennis, S., Chami, F., Chami, N., Bouchikhi, T., & Remmal, A. (2004). Surface alteration of Saccharomyces cerevisiae induced by thymol and eugenol. Letters in Applied Microbiology, 38(6), 454-458.

Chami, N., Bennis, S., Chami, F., Aboussekhra, A., & Remmal, A. (2005). Study of anticandidal activity of carvacrol and eugenol in vitro and in vivo. Molecular Oral Microbiology, 20(2), 106-111.

Leuschner, R. G., & Ielsch, V. (2003). Antimicrobial effects of garlic, clove and red hot chilli on Listeria monocytogenes in broth model systems and soft cheese. International journal of food sciences and nutrition, 54(2), 127-133.

Miyazawa, M., & Hisama, M. (2003). Antimutagenic activity of phenylpropanoids from clove (Syzygium aromaticum). Journal of Agricultural and Food Chemistry, 51(22), 6413-6422.

Somova, L. O., Nadar, A., Rammanan, P., & Shode, F. O. (2003).

Cardiovascular, antihyperlipidemic and antioxidant effects of oleanolic and ursolic acids in experimental hypertension. Phytomedicine, 10(2-3), 115-121.

Guynot, M. E., Ramos, A. J., Seto, L., Purroy, P., Sanchis, V., & Marin, S. (2003). Antifungal activity of volatile compounds generated by essential oils against fungi commonly causing deterioration of bakery products. Journal of Applied Microbiology, 94(5), 893-899.

Chami, F., Chami, N., Bennis, S., Trouillas, J., & Remmal, A. (2004). Evaluation of carvacrol and eugenol as prophylaxis and treatment of vaginal candidiasis in an immunosuppressed rat model. Journal of Antimicrobial Chemotherapy, 54(5), 909-914.

Alqareer, A., Alyahya, A., & Andersson, L. (2006). The effect of clove and benzocaine versus placebo as topical anesthetics. Journal of dentistry, 34(10), 747-750.

Park, B. S., Song, Y. S., Yee, S. B., Lee, B. G., Seo, S. Y., Park, Y. C., ... & Yoo, Y. H. (2005). Phospho-ser 15-p53 translocates into mitochondria and interacts with Bcl-2 and Bcl-xL in eugenol-induced apoptosis. Apoptosis, 10(1), 193-200.

Feng, J., & Lipton, J. M. (1987). Eugenol: antipyretic activity in rabbits. Neuropharmacology, 26(12), 1775-1778.

Damiani, C. E. N., Rossoni, L. V., & Vassallo, D. V. (2003). Vasorelaxant effects of eugenol on rat thoracic aorta. Vascular pharmacology, 40(1), 59-66.

Kumari, M. R. (1991). Modulatory influences of clove (Caryophyllus aromaticus, L) on hepatic detoxification systems and bone marrow genotoxicity in male Swiss albino mice. Cancer letters, 60(1), 67-73.

Friedman, M., Henika, P. R., Levin, C. E., & Mandrell, R. E. (2004). Antibacterial activities of plant essential oils and their components against

Escherichia coli O157: H7 and Salmonella enterica in apple juice. Journal of agricultural and food chemistry, 52(19), 6042-6048.

Schecter, A., Lucier, G. W., Cunningham, M. L., Abdo, K. M., Blumenthal, G., Silver, A. G., ... & Stanfill, S. B. (2004). Human consumption of methyleugenol and its elimination from serum. Environmental health perspectives, 112(6), 678.

Kim, S. S., Oh, O. J., Min, H. Y., Park, E. J., Kim, Y., Park, H. J., ... & Lee, S. K. (2003). Eugenol suppresses cyclooxygenase-2 expression in lipopolysaccharide-stimulated mouse macrophage RAW264. 7 cells. Life sciences, 73(3), 337-348.

CHAPTER Marijuana, fiber, intoxicant and medicine

Hall, W., & Degenhardt, L. (2009). Adverse health effects of non-medical cannabis use. The Lancet, 374(9698), 1383-1391.

Hall, W. (2009). The adverse health effects of cannabis use: what are they, and what are their implications for policy?. International Journal of drug policy, 20(6), 458-466.

Pew Research Center, April 2014, "America's Changing Drug Policy Landscape"; http://www.people-press.org/files/legacy-pdf/04-02-14%20 Drug%20Policy%20Release.pdf.

Thomas, G., Kloner, R. A., & Rezkalla, S. (2014). Adverse cardiovascular, cerebrovascular, and peripheral vascular effects of marijuana inhalation: what cardiologists need to know. American Journal of Cardiology, 113(1), 187-190.

Lopez-Quintero, C., de los Cobos, J. P., Hasin, D. S., Okuda, M., Wang, S., Grant, B. F., & Blanco, C. (2011). Probability and predictors of transition from first use to dependence on nicotine, alcohol, cannabis, and cocaine: results of the National Epidemiologic Survey on Alcohol and Related

Conditions (NESARC). Drug & Alcohol Dependence, 115(1), 120-130.

Meier, M. H., Caspi, A., Ambler, A., Harrington, H., Houts, R., Keefe, R. S., ... & Moffitt, T. E. (2012). Persistent cannabis users show neuropsychological decline from childhood to midlife. Proceedings of the National Academy of Sciences, 109(40), E2657-E2664.

Meier, M. H., Caspi, A., Ambler, A., Harrington, H., Houts, R., Keefe, R. S., ... & Moffitt, T. E. (2012). Persistent cannabis users show neuropsychological decline from childhood to midlife. Proceedings of the National Academy of Sciences, 109(40), E2657-E2664.

Crean, R. D., Crane, N. A., & Mason, B. J. (2011). An evidence based review of acute and long-term effects of cannabis use on executive cognitive functions. Journal of addiction medicine, 5(1), 1.

Lynskey, M., & Hall, W. (2000). The effects of adolescent cannabis use on educational attainment: A review. Addiction, 95(11), 1621-1630.

Bray, J. W., Zarkin, G. A., Ringwalt, C., & Qi, J. (2000). The relationship between marijuana initiation and dropping out of high school. Health Economics, 9(1), 9-18.

Tortoriello, G., Morris, C. V., Alpar, A., Fuzik, J., Shirran, S. L., Calvigioni, D., ... & Courtney, M. (2014). Miswiring the brain: Δ9-tetrahydrocannabinol disrupts cortical development by inducing an SCG10/stathmin-2 degradation pathway. The EMBO journal, 33(7), 668-685.

Casadio, P., Fernandes, C., Murray, R. M., & Di Forti, M. (2011). Cannabis use in young people: the risk for schizophrenia. Neuroscience & Biobehavioral Reviews, 35(8), 1779-1787.

Tashkin, D. P. (2013). Effects of marijuana smoking on the lung. Annals of the American Thoracic Society, 10(3), 239-247.

Owen, K. P., Sutter, M. E., & Albertson, T. E. (2014). Marijuana: respiratory tract effects. Clinical reviews in allergy & immunology, 46(1), 65-81.

Hashibe, M., Morgenstern, H., Cui, Y., Tashkin, D. P., Zhang, Z. F., Cozen, W., ... & Greenland, S. (2006). Marijuana use and the risk of lung and upper aerodigestive tract cancers: results of a population-based case-control study. Cancer Epidemiology and Prevention Biomarkers, 15(10), 1829-1834.

Lacson, J. C. A., Carroll, J. D., Tuazon, E., Castelao, E. J., Bernstein, L., & Cortessis, V. K. (2012). Population-based case-control study of recreational drug use and testis cancer risk confirms an association between marijuana use and nonseminoma risk. Cancer, 118(21), 5374-5383.

Daling, J. R., Doody, D. R., Sun, X., Trabert, B. L., Weiss, N. S., Chen, C., ... & Schwartz, S. M. (2009). Association of marijuana use and the incidence of testicular germ cell tumors. Cancer, 115(6), 1215-1223.

CHAPTER GINSENG research supported medicinal properties

Reay, J. L., Kennedy, D. O., & Scholey, A. B. (2016). Effects of Panax ginseng, consumed with and without glucose, on blood glucose levels and cognitive performance during sustained 'mentally demanding'tasks. Journal of Psychopharmacology, 20(6), 771-781.

Kennedy, D. O., Scholey, A. B., & Wesnes, K. A. (2001). Differential, dose dependent changes in cognitive performance following acute administration of a Ginkgo biloba/Panax ginseng combination to healthy young volunteers. Nutritional neuroscience, 4(5), 399-412.

Wesnes, K. W., Faleni, R. A., Hefting, N. R., & Hoogsteen, G. (1997). The cognitive, subjective, and physical effects of a ginkgo biloba/ panax ginseng combination in healthy volunteers with neurasthenic complaints. Psychopharmacology Bulletin, 33(4), 677.

Hartley, D. E., Elsabagh, S., & File, S. E. (2004). Gincosan (a combination of Ginkgo biloba and Panax ginseng): the effects on mood and cognition of 6 and 12 weeks' treatment in post-menopausal women. Nutritional neuroscience, 7(5-6), 325-333.

Kennedy, D. O., Haskell, C. F., Wesnes, K. A., & Scholey, A. B. (2004). Improved cognitive performance in human volunteers following administration of guarana (Paullinia cupana) extract: comparison and interaction with Panax ginseng.
Pharmacology Biochemistry and Behavior, 79(3), 401-411.

Gurley, B. J., Gardner, S. F., Hubbard, M. A., Williams, D. K., Gentry, W. B., Cui, Y., & Ang, C. Y. (2005). Clinical assessment of effects of botanical supplementation on cytochrome P450 phenotypes in the elderly. Drugs & aging, 22(6), 525-539.

Ito, T. Y., Trant, A. S., & Polan, M. L. (2001). A double-blind placebo-controlled study of ArginMax, a nutritional supplement for enhancement of female sexual function. Journal of Sex &Marital Therapy, 27(5), 541-549.

Liu, P., Xu, Y., Yin, H., Wang, J., Chen, K., & Li, Y. (2005). Developmental toxicity research of ginsenoside Rb1 using a whole mouse embryo culture model. Birth Defects Research Part B: Developmental and Reproductive Toxicology, 74(2), 207-209.

Liu, P., Yin, H., Xu, Y., Zhang, Z., Chen, K., & Li, Y. (2006). Effects of ginsenoside Rg1 on postimplantation rat and mouse embryos cultured in vitro. Toxicology in vitro, 20(2), 234-238.

Lee, Y. H., Lee, B. K., Choi, Y. J., Yoon, I. K., Chang, B. C., & Gwak, H. S. (2010). Interaction between warfarin and Korean red ginseng in patients with cardiac valve replacement. International journal of cardiology, 145(2), 275-276.

Engels, H. J., Fahlman, M. M., & Wirth, J. C. (2003). Effects of ginseng on secretory IgA, performance, and recovery from interval exercise. Medicine and science in sports and exercise, 35(4), 690-696.

Onanong Kulaputana, M. D. (2007). Ginseng supplementation does not change lactate threshold and physical performances in physically active Thai men. J Med Assoc Thai, 90(6), 1172-9.

Cho, S., Won, C. H., Lee, D. H., Lee, M. J., Lee, S., So, S. H., ... & Chung, J. H. (2009). Red ginseng root extract mixed with Torilus fructus and Corni fructus improves facial wrinkles and increases type I procollagen synthesis in human skin: a randomized, double-blind, placebo-controlled study. Journal of medicinal food, 12(6), 1252-1259.

Kim, J. H., Park, C. Y., & Lee, S. J. (2006). Effects of Sun Ginseng on subjective quality of life in cancer patients: a double-blind, placebo-controlled pilot trial. Journal of clinical pharmacy and therapeutics, 31(4), 331-334.

Ni, H. X., Yu, N. J., & Yang, X. H. (2010). The study of ginsenoside on PPARγ expression of mononuclear macrophage in type 2 diabetes. Molecular biology reports, 37(6), 2975-2979.

Shin, S. K., Kwon, J. H., Jeong, Y. J., Jeon, S. M., Choi, J. Y., & Choi, M. S. (2011). Supplementation of cheonggukjang and red ginseng cheonggukjang can improve plasma lipid profile and fasting blood glucose concentration in subjects with impaired fasting glucose. Journal of medicinal food, 14(1-2), 108-113.

Kim, T. H., Jeon, S. H., Hahn, E. J., Paek, K. Y., Park, J. K., Youn, N. Y., & Lee, H. L. (2009). Effects of tissue-cultured mountain ginseng (Panax ginseng CA Meyer) extract on male patients with erectile dysfunction. Asian journal of andrology, 11(3), 356.

Jang, D. J., Lee, M. S., Shin, B. C., Lee, Y. C., & Ernst, E. (2008). Red ginseng for treating erectile dysfunction: a systematic review. British journal of clinical pharmacology, 66(4), 444-450.

Han, K. H., Choe, S. C., Kim, H. S., Sohn, D. W., Nam, K. Y., Oh, B. H., … & Lee, Y. W. (1998). Effect of red ginseng on blood pressure in patients with essential hypertension and white coat hypertension. The American journal of Chinese medicine, 26(02), 199-209.

Oh, K. J., Chae, M. J., Lee, H. S., Hong, H. D., & Park, K. (2010). Effects of Korean red ginseng on sexual arousal in menopausal women: Placebo-controlled, double-blind crossover clinical study. The journal of sexual medicine, 7(4pt1), 1469-1477.

Sung, H., Jung, Y. S., & Cho, Y. K. (2009). Beneficial effects of a combination of Korean red ginseng and highly active antiretroviral therapy in human immunodeficiency virus type 1-infected patients. Clinical and Vaccine Immunology, 16(8), 1127-1131.

Lee, J. S., Kwon, K. A., Jung, H. S., Kim, J. H., & Hahm, K. B. (2009). Korea red ginseng on Helicobacter pylori-induced halitosis: newer therapeutic strategy and a plausible
mechanism. Digestion, 80(3), 192-199.

Le Gal, M., Cathebras, P., & Strüby, K. (1996). Pharmaton capsules in the treatment of functional fatigue: A double-blind study versus placebo evaluated by a new methodology. Phytotherapy Research, 10(1), 49-53.

Yun, T. K., Zheng, S., Choi, S. Y., Cai, S. R., Lee, Y. S., Liu, X. Y., … & Park, K. Y. (2010). Non–organ-specific preventive effect of long-term administration of Korean Red Ginseng extract on incidence of human cancers. Journal of medicinal food, 13(3), 489-494.

Mateo-Carrasco, H., Gálvez-Contreras, M. C., Fernández-Ginés, F. D., & Nguyen, T. V. (2012). Elevated liver enzymes resulting from an interaction between Raltegravir and Panax ginseng: a case report and brief review.

Lee, S. T., Chu, K., Sim, J. Y., Heo, J. H., & Kim, M. (2008). Panax ginseng enhances cognitive performance in Alzheimer disease. Alzheimer Disease & Associated Disorders, 22(3), 222-226.

Heo, J. H., Lee, S. T., Chu, K., Oh, M. J., Park, H. J., Shim, J. Y., & Kim, M. (2008). An open-label trial of Korean red ginseng as an adjuvant treatment for cognitive impairment in patients with Alzheimer's disease. European Journal of Neurology, 15(8), 865-868.

Reay, J. L., Kennedy, D. O., & Scholey, A. B. (2006). Effects of Panax ginseng, consumed with and without glucose, on blood glucose levels and cognitive performance during sustained 'mentally demanding'tasks. Journal of Psychopharmacology, 20(6), 771-781.

Reay, J. L., Kennedy, D. O., & Scholey, A. B. (2005). Single doses of Panax ginseng (G115) reduce blood glucose levels and improve cognitive performance during sustained mental activity. Journal of Psychopharmacology, 19(4), 357-365.

Neri, M., Andermarcher, E., Pradelli, J. M., & Salvioli, G. (1995). Influence of a double blind pharmacological trial on two domains of well-being in subjects with age associated memory impairment. Archives of gerontology and geriatrics, 21(3), 241-252.

Reay, J. L., Scholey, A. B., & Kennedy, D. O. (2010). Panax ginseng (G115) improves aspects of working memory performance and subjective ratings of calmness in healthy young adults. Human Psychopharmacology: Clinical and Experimental, 25(6), 462-471.

Smith, M., Lin, K. M., & Zheng, Y. P. (2001). Piii-89 An Open Trial Of Nifedipine-herb Interactions: Nifedipine With St. John's Wort, Ginseng Or Ginko Biloba. Clinical Pharmacology & Therapeutics, 69(2), P86.

An, X., Zhang, A. L., Yang, A. W., Lin, L., Wu, D., Guo, X., ... & Xue, C. C. (2011). Oral ginseng formulae for stable chronic obstructive pulmonary disease: a systematic review. Respiratory medicine, 105(2), 165-176.

Reeds, D. N., Patterson, B. W., Okunade, A., Holloszy, J. O., Polonsky, K. S., & Klein, S. (2011). Ginseng and ginsenoside Re do not improve β-cell function or insulin sensitivity in overweight and obese subjects with impaired glucose tolerance or diabetes. Diabetes care, 34(5), 1071-1076.

Dasgupta, A., Tso, G., & Wells, A. (2008). Effect of Asian ginseng, Siberian ginseng, and Indian ayurvedic medicine Ashwagandha on serum digoxin measurement by Digoxin III, a new digoxin immunoassay. Journal of clinical laboratory analysis, 22(4), 295-301.

Cui, Y., Shu, X. O., Gao, Y. T., Cai, H., Tao, M. H., & Zheng, W. (2006). Association of ginseng use with survival and quality of life among breast cancer patients. American journal of epidemiology, 163(7), 645-653.

Kabalak, A. A., Soyal, O. B., Urfalioglu, A., Saracoglu, F., & Gogus, N. (2004). Menometrorrhagia and tachyarrhythmia after using oral and topical ginseng. Journal of Women's Health, 13(7), 830-833.

Kim, S. H., Park, K. S., Chang, M. J., & Sung, J. H. (2005). Effects of Panax ginseng extract on exercise-induced oxidative stress. Journal of Sports Medicine and Physical Fitness, 45(2), 178.

Keum, Y. S., Park, K. K., Lee, J. M., Chun, K. S., Park, J. H., Lee, S. K., … & Surh, Y. J. (2000). Antioxidant and anti-tumor promoting activities of the methanol extract of heat-processed ginseng. Cancer letters, 150(1), 41-48.

Lee, Y. J., Jin, Y. R., Lim, W. C., Park, W. K., Cho, J. Y., Jang, S., & Lee, S. K. (2003). Ginsenoside-R b1 acts as a weak phytoestrogen in MCF-7 human breast cancer cells. Archives of pharmacal research, 26(1), 58-63.

Wiklund, I. K., Mattsson, L. A., Lindgren, R., & Limoni, C. (1999). Effects of a standardized ginseng extract on quality of life and physiological parameters in symptomatic postmenopausal women: a double-blind, placebo-controlled trial. Swedish Alternative Medicine Group. International journal of clinical pharmacology research, 19(3), 89-99.

Hong, B., Ji, Y. H., Hong, J. H., Nam, K. Y., & Ahn, T. Y. (2002). A double-blind crossover study evaluating the efficacy of Korean red ginseng in patients with erectile dysfunction: a preliminary report. The Journal of urology, 168(5), 2070-2073.

Ng, T. B., & Wang, H. (2001). Panaxagin, a new protein from Chinese ginseng possesses anti-fungal, anti-viral, translation-inhibiting and ribonuclease activities. Life sciences, 68(7), 739-749.

Ellis, J. M., & Reddy, P. (2002). Effects of Panax ginseng on quality of life. Annals of Pharmacotherapy, 36(3), 375-379.

Scholey, A. B., & Kennedy, D. O. (2002). Acute, dose-dependent cognitive effects of Ginkgo biloba, Panax ginseng and their combination in healthy young volunteers: differential interactions with cognitive demand. Human Psychopharmacology: Clinical and Experimental, 17(1), 35-44.

Vuksan, V., Stavro, M. P., Sievenpiper, J. L., Beljan-Zdravkovic, U., Leiter, L. A., Josse, R. G., & Xu, Z. H. E. N. G. (2000). Similar postprandial glycemic reductions with escalation of dose and administration time of American ginseng in type 2 diabetes. Diabetes Care, 23(9), 1221-1226.

Caron, M. F., Hotsko, A. L., Robertson, S., Mandybur, L., Kluger, J., & White, C. M. (2002). Electrocardiographic and hemodynamic effects of Panax ginseng. Annals of Pharmacotherapy, 36(5), 758-763.

Ding, D. Z., Shen, T. K., & Cui, Y. Z. (1995). Effects of red ginseng on the congestive heart failure and its mechanism. Zhongguo Zhong xi yi jie he za zhi Zhongguo Zhongxiyi jiehe zazhi= Chinese journal of integrated traditional and Western medicine, 15(6), 325-327.

Lee, B. M., Lee, S. K., & Kim, H. S. (1998). Inhibition of oxidative DNA damage, 8-OHdG, and carbonyl contents in smokers treated with antioxidants (vitamin E, vitamin C, β-carotene and red ginseng). Cancer letters, 132(1), 219-227.

KASE, Y., Saitoh, K., Ishige, A., & KOMATSU, Y. (1998). Mechanisms by which Hange-shashin-to reduces prostaglandin E2 levels. Biological and Pharmaceutical Bulletin, 21(12), 1277-1281.

Hiai, S., YOKOYAMA, H., OURA, H., & YANO, S. (1979). Stimulation of pituitary-adrenocortical system by ginseng saponin. Endocrinologia japonica, 26(6), 661-665.

Song, Z., Kharazmi, A., Wu, H., Faber, V., Moser, C., Johansen, H. K., … & Høiby, N. (1998). Effects of ginseng treatment on neutrophil chemiluminescence and immunoglobulin G subclasses in a rat model of chronic Pseudomonas aeruginosa pneumonia. Clinical and diagnostic laboratory immunology, 5(6), 882-887.

Ryu, S. J., & Chien, Y. Y. (1995). Ginseng-associated cerebral arteritis. Neurology, 45(4), 829-830.

Hopkins, M. P., Androff, L., & Benninghoff, A. S. (1988). Ginseng face cream and unexplained vaginal bleeding. American Journal of Obstetrics & Gynecology, 159(5), 1121-1122.

Made in the USA
Monee, IL
19 August 2022

11874259R00151